IMPLEMENTATION OF
Lung Cancer Screening

Proceedings of a Workshop

Erin Balogh, Margie Patlak, and Sharyl J. Nass, *Rapporteurs*

National Cancer Policy Forum

Board on Health Care Services

Health and Medicine Division

The National Academies of
SCIENCES · ENGINEERING · MEDICINE

THE NATIONAL ACADEMIES PRESS
Washington, DC
www.nap.edu

THE NATIONAL ACADEMIES PRESS 500 Fifth Street, NW Washington, DC 20001

This project was supported by Contract No. 200-2011-38807 (Task Order No. 0051) and Contract No. HHSN263201200074I (Task Order No. HHSN26300052) with the Centers for Disease Control and Prevention and the National Cancer Institute/ National Institutes of Health, respectively, and by the American Association for Cancer Research, American Cancer Society, American College of Radiology, American Society for Radiation Oncology, American Society of Clinical Oncology, American Society of Hematology, Association of American Cancer Institutes, AstraZeneca, Bristol-Myers Squibb, Cancer Support Community, CEO Roundtable on Cancer, Helsinn Healthcare SA, LIVESTRONG Foundation, National Comprehensive Cancer Network, Novartis Oncology, Oncology Nursing Society, and Pfizer Inc. Any opinions, findings, conclusions, or recommendations expressed in this publication do not necessarily reflect the views of any organization or agency that provided support for the project.

International Standard Book Number-13: 978-0-309-45132-1
International Standard Book Number-10: 0-309-45132-9
Digital Object Identifier https://doi.org/10.172216/23680

Additional copies of this publication are available for sale from the National Academies Press, 500 Fifth Street, NW, Keck 360, Washington, DC 20001; (800) 624-6242 or (202) 334-3313; http://www.nap.edu.

Printed in the United States of America

Suggested citation: National Academies of Sciences, Engineering, and Medicine. 2017. *Implementation of lung cancer screening: Proceedings of a workshop*. Washington, DC: The National Academies Press. doi: https://doi.org/10.172216/23680.

The National Academies of

SCIENCES · ENGINEERING · MEDICINE

The **National Academy of Sciences** was established in 1863 by an Act of Congress, signed by President Lincoln, as a private, nongovernmental institution to advise the nation on issues related to science and technology. Members are elected by their peers for outstanding contributions to research. Dr. Marcia McNutt is president.

The **National Academy of Engineering** was established in 1964 under the charter of the National Academy of Sciences to bring the practices of engineering to advising the nation. Members are elected by their peers for extraordinary contributions to engineering. Dr. C. D. Mote, Jr., is president.

The **National Academy of Medicine** (formerly the Institute of Medicine) was established in 1970 under the charter of the National Academy of Sciences to advise the nation on medical and health issues. Members are elected by their peers for distinguished contributions to medicine and health. Dr. Victor J. Dzau is president.

The three Academies work together as the **National Academies of Sciences, Engineering, and Medicine** to provide independent, objective analysis and advice to the nation and conduct other activities to solve complex problems and inform public policy decisions. The National Academies also encourage education and research, recognize outstanding contributions to knowledge, and increase public understanding in matters of science, engineering, and medicine.

Learn more about the National Academies of Sciences, Engineering, and Medicine at **www.national-academies.org**.

The National Academies of

SCIENCES • ENGINEERING • MEDICINE

Reports document the evidence-based consensus of an authoring committee of experts. Reports typically include findings, conclusions, and recommendations based on information gathered by the committee and committee deliberations. Reports are peer reviewed and are approved by the National Academies of Sciences, Engineering, and Medicine.

Proceedings chronicle the presentations and discussions at a workshop, symposium, or other convening event. The statements and opinions contained in proceedings are those of the participants and have not been endorsed by other participants, the planning committee, or the National Academies of Sciences, Engineering, and Medicine.

For information about other products and activities of the National Academies, please visit nationalacademies.org/whatwedo.

WORKSHOP PLANNING COMMITTEE[1]

GRETA MASSETTI (*Chair*), Associate Director for Science, Division of Cancer Prevention and Control, Centers for Disease Control and Prevention

LORI HOFFMAN HŌGG, Veterans Health Administration National Oncology Clinical Advisor and Program Manager, Prevention Policy, Department of Veterans Affairs

SAMIR N. KHLEIF, Professor of Medicine, Biochemistry, Molecular Biology, and Graduate Studies, Augusta University

BARNETT KRAMER, Director, Division of Cancer Prevention, National Cancer Institute

LEE M. KRUG, Disease Area Head, Lung and Head & Neck Cancer, Immuno-Oncology, Bristol-Myers Squibb

CHRISTOPHER S. LATHAN, Assistant Professor of Medicine, Harvard Medical School; Director, Cancer Care Equity, Dana-Farber Cancer Institute

JENNIFER A. PIETENPOL, Director, Vanderbilt-Ingraham Cancer Center; Executive Vice President for Research, Vanderbilt University Medical Center; and Benjamin F. Byrd, Jr. Professor of Oncology, Vanderbilt University

YA-CHEN TINA SHIH, Professor of Health Economics, Chief, Section of Cancer Economics and Policy, Department of Health Services Research, University of Texas MD Anderson Cancer Center

ROBERT SMITH, Vice President, Cancer Screening, American Cancer Society

JAMIE L. STUDTS, Associate Professor, Department of Behavioral Science, University of Kentucky College of Medicine; Director, Behavioral & Community-Based Research Shared Resource Facility, Markey Cancer Center

DANIEL SULLIVAN, Professor Emeritus, Department of Radiology, Duke University School of Medicine

[1] The National Academies of Sciences, Engineering, and Medicine's planning committees are solely responsible for organizing the workshop, identifying topics, and choosing speakers. The responsibility for the published Proceedings of a Workshop rests with the workshop rapporteurs and the institution.

ROBERT J. VOLK, Professor, Department of Health Services Research, Division of Cancer Prevention and Population Sciences, University of Texas MD Anderson Cancer Center

Project Staff

SHARYL J. NASS, Director, National Cancer Policy Forum
ERIN BALOGH, Senior Program Officer
CYNDI TRANG, Research Assistant
PATRICK ROSS, Research Assistant (*until July 2016*)

NATIONAL CANCER POLICY FORUM[1]

[1] The National Academies of Sciences, Engineering, and Medicine's forums and roundtables do not issue, review, or approve individual documents. The responsibility for the published Proceedings of a Workshop rests with the workshop rapporteurs and the institution.

GEORGE D. DEMETRI, Professor of Medicine, Harvard Medical School; Director, Ludwig Center; Senior Vice President for Experimental Therapeutics, Dana-Farber Cancer Institute; Associate Director for Clinical Sciences, Dana-Farber/Harvard Cancer Center

JAMES H. DOROSHOW, Deputy Director for Clinical and Translational Research, National Cancer Institute

JOHN FRIEND II, Senior Vice President, Helsinn Therapeutics

LORI HOFFMAN HŌGG, Veterans Health Administration National Oncology Clinical Advisor and Program Manager, Prevention Policy, Department of Veterans Affairs

LINDA HOUSE, President, Cancer Support Community

HEDVIG HRICAK, Chair, Department of Radiology, Memorial Sloan Kettering Cancer Center

LISA KENNEDY SHELDON, Chief Clinical Officer, Oncology Nursing Society; Editor, *Clinical Journal of Oncology Nursing*

SAMIR N. KHLEIF, Professor of Medicine, Biochemistry, Molecular Biology, and Graduate Studies, Augusta University

RONALD M. KLINE, Medical Officer, Patient Care Models Group, Center for Medicare & Medicaid Innovation, Centers for Medicare & Medicaid Services

LEE M. KRUG, Disease Area Head, Lung and Head & Neck Cancer, Immuno-Oncology, Bristol-Myers Squibb

RICHARD A. LARSON, Professor of Medicine and Director, Hematologic Malignancies Clinical Research Program, The University of Chicago Comprehensive Cancer Center

MICHELLE M. LE BEAU, Arthur and Marian Edelstein Professor of Medicine and Director, The University of Chicago Comprehensive Cancer Center

GRETA MASSETTI, Associate Director for Science, Division of Cancer Prevention and Control, Centers for Disease Control and Prevention

DANIEL R. MASYS, Affiliate Professor, Biomedical and Health Informatics, University of Washington School of Medicine

MARTIN J. MURPHY, Chief Executive Officer, CEO Roundtable on Cancer

LOYCE PACE, Executive Director, Global Health Council (LIVESTRONG Representative)

RICHARD PAZDUR, Director, Oncology Center of Excellence; Acting Director, Office of Hematology and Oncology Products, Food and Drug Administration

STEVEN PIANTADOSI, Phase One Foundation Endowed Chair and Director, Samuel Oschin Comprehensive Cancer Institute, Cedars-Sinai Medical Center

JENNIFER A. PIETENPOL, Director, Vanderbilt-Ingraham Cancer Center; Executive Vice President for Research, Vanderbilt University Medical Center; and Benjamin F. Byrd, Jr. Professor of Oncology, Vanderbilt University

MACE L. ROTHENBERG, Chief Development Officer, Oncology, Pfizer Global Product Development, Pfizer Inc.

RICHARD L. SCHILSKY, Senior Vice President and Chief Medical Officer, American Society of Clinical Oncology

DEBORAH SCHRAG, Chief, Division of Population Sciences, Professor of Medicine, Department of Medical Oncology, Harvard Medical School, Dana-Farber Cancer Institute

YA-CHEN TINA SHIH, Professor of Health Economics, Chief, Section of Cancer Economics and Policy, Department of Health Services Research, University of Texas MD Anderson Cancer Center

ELLEN V. SIGAL, Chair and Founder, Friends of Cancer Research

RALPH WEICHSELBAUM, Daniel K. Ludwig Professor and Chair, Department of Radiation; Oncology and Cellular Director, Ludwig Center for Metastasis Research, The University of Chicago Medical Center

GEORGE J. WEINER, President, Association of American Cancer Institutes; C.E. Block Chair of Cancer Research, Professor of Internal Medicine, and Director, Holden Comprehensive Cancer Center, University of Iowa

RICHARD WOODMAN, Senior Vice President and Head, North America Oncology Clinical Development & Medical Affairs, Novartis Pharmaceuticals Corporation

WENDY WOODWARD, Associate Professor and Section Chief of Clinical Breast Radiation, Department of Radiation Oncology, University of Texas MD Anderson Cancer Center

National Cancer Policy Forum Staff

SHARYL J. NASS, Forum Director and Director, Board on Health Care Services
ERIN BALOGH, Senior Program Officer
SYLARA MARIE CRUZ, Senior Program Assistant
MATINA KAKALIS, Summer Intern (*May-July 2016*)
KIMBERLY MAXFIELD, Mirzayan Science and Technology Policy Fellow (*January-May 2016*)
PATRICK ROSS, Research Assistant (*until July 2016*)
CYNDI TRANG, Research Assistant
PATRICK BURKE, Financial Officer

Reviewers

This Proceedings of a Workshop has been reviewed in draft form by individuals chosen for their diverse perspectives and technical expertise. The purpose of this independent review is to provide candid and critical comments that will assist the institution in making its published Proceedings of a Workshop as sound as possible and to ensure that the Proceedings of a Workshop meets institutional standards for objectivity, evidence, and responsiveness to the study charge. The review comments and draft manuscript remain confidential to protect the integrity of the process. We wish to thank the following individuals for their review of this Proceedings of a Workshop:

MICHAEL K. GOULD, Kaiser Permanente
ELLA KAZEROONI, University of Michigan
MICHAEL L. LeFEVRE, University of Missouri
PETER MAZZONE, Cleveland Clinic
IDE MILLS, Patient Advocate

Although the reviewers listed above have provided many constructive comments and suggestions, they did not see the final draft of the Proceedings of a Workshop before its release. The review of this Proceedings of a Workshop was overseen by **SUSAN J. CURRY,** University of Iowa. She was responsible for making certain that an independent examination of this Proceedings of a Workshop was carried out in accordance with institutional procedures and that all review comments were carefully considered. Responsibility for the final content of this Proceedings of a Workshop rests entirely with the rapporteurs and the institution.

IN MEMORIAM

This Proceedings of a Workshop is dedicated to Dr. Gregory Curt, an accomplished physician and scientist, a valued member of the National Cancer Policy Forum, and an irreplaceable colleague and friend.

Acknowledgments

Support from the many annual sponsors of the National Academies of Sciences, Engineering, and Medicine's National Cancer Policy Forum is crucial to the work of the Forum. Federal sponsors include the Centers for Disease Control and Prevention and the National Cancer Institute/National Institutes of Health. Non-federal sponsors include the American Association for Cancer Research, American Cancer Society, American College of Radiology, American Society for Radiation Oncology, American Society of Clinical Oncology, American Society of Hematology, Association of American Cancer Institutes, AstraZeneca, Bristol-Myers Squibb, Cancer Support Community, CEO Roundtable on Cancer, Helsinn Healthcare SA, LIVESTRONG Foundation, National Comprehensive Cancer Network, Novartis Oncology, Oncology Nursing Society, and Pfizer Inc.

The Forum wishes to express its gratitude to the expert speakers whose presentations helped examine the policy and implementation issues in lung cancer screening. The Forum also wishes to thank the members of the planning committee for their work in developing an excellent workshop agenda.

Contents

Boxes, Figures, and Tables

BOXES

FIGURES

TABLES

Acronyms and Abbreviations

AAFP	American Academy of Family Physicians
AATS	American Association for Thoracic Surgery
ACA	Patient Protection and Affordable Care Act
ACCP	American College of Chest Physicians
ACR	American College of Radiology
ACS	American Cancer Society
AHRQ	Agency for Healthcare Research and Quality
ALA	American Lung Association
ASCO	American Society of Clinical Oncology
ATS	American Thoracic Society
BI-RADS	Breast Imaging Reporting and Data System
CDC	Centers for Disease Control and Prevention
CMS	Centers for Medicare & Medicaid Services
COPD	chronic obstructive pulmonary disorder
CT	computed tomography
DANTE	Detection and Screening of Early Lung Cancer by Novel Imaging Technology and Molecular Essays
DLCST	Danish Lung Cancer Screening Trial

EMR	electronic medical record
FDA	Food and Drug Administration
GOLF	Groupe d'Oncologie de Langue Française
HEDIS	Healthcare Effectiveness Data and Information Set
IASLC	International Association for the Study of Lung Cancer
I-ELCAP	International-Early Lung Cancer Action Program
IFCT	French Cooperative Thoracic Intergroup
IPDAS	International Patient Decision Aids Standards Collaboration
LDCT	low-dose computed tomography
Lung-RADS	ACR Lung Imaging Reporting and Data System
MEDCAC	Medicare Evidence Development and Coverage Advisory Committee
NCCN	National Comprehensive Cancer Network
NCD	national coverage determination
NCI	National Cancer Institute
NELSON	Nederlands-Leuvens Longkanker Screenings Onderzoek
NLST	National Lung Screening Trial
PET	positron emission tomography
PLCO	Prostate, Lung, Colorectal, and Ovarian Cancer Screening Trial
PROSPR	Population-based Research Optimizing Screening through Personalized Regimens
QALY	quality-adjusted life year
USPSTF	U.S. Preventive Services Task Force
VA	Department of Veterans Affairs

Proceedings of a Workshop

INTRODUCTION[1]

The public health burden from lung cancer is substantial: it is the second most commonly diagnosed cancer and the leading cause of cancer-related deaths in the United States (ACS, 2016), said Greta Massetti, associate director for science at the Centers for Disease Control and Prevention's (CDC's) Division of Cancer Prevention and Control. Each year, more people die from lung cancer than from colon, breast, and prostate cancers combined; in addition, the 5-year relative survival rate of patients with lung cancer is only 17 percent (ACS, 2016). More than half of people with lung cancer are diagnosed with metastatic disease, in which the cancer has spread to distant organs or lymph nodes (NCI, 2016c). Symptoms often do not appear until the disease is advanced, and the symptoms also can be mistaken for other health conditions (ACS, 2016). And even for localized lung cancer, the 5-year relative survival rate is low compared to many other common cancers

[1] The planning committee's role was limited to planning the workshop. The Proceedings of a Workshop has been prepared by the rapporteurs as a factual account of what occurred at the workshop. Statements, recommendations, and opinions expressed are those of individual presenters and participants and have not been endorsed or verified by the National Academies of Sciences, Engineering, and Medicine. They should not be construed as reflecting any group consensus.

(55 percent for lung cancer versus more than 90 percent for breast, cervical, and colorectal cancers), said Massetti (ACS, 2016).

Given the individual and population health burden of lung cancer, especially when it is diagnosed at later stages, Massetti noted that there has been a push to develop and implement screening strategies for early detection. The National Lung Screening Trial (NLST) evaluated the effectiveness of annual screening with low-dose computed tomography (LDCT) to reduce lung cancer mortality among individuals at high risk for lung cancer. Results from the trial demonstrated a 20 percent reduction in mortality from lung cancer for patients screened with LDCT (The National Lung Screening Trial Research Team et al., 2011). In 2013, the U.S. Preventive Services Task Force (USPSTF) recommended annual lung cancer screening with LDCT for asymptomatic persons at high risk[2] of developing lung cancer. For LDCT screening, the USPSTF assigned a grade B recommendation, which is defined as a "high certainty that the net benefit is moderate or there is moderate certainty that the net benefit is moderate to substantial" (USPSTF, 2016b). Provisions of the Patient Protection and Affordable Care Act (ACA) require some private insurers to cover USPSTF-recommended preventive health services with a grade A or B without patient cost sharing.[3] In addition, the Centers for Medicare & Medicaid Services (CMS) issued a Medicare national coverage determination for lung cancer screening, including counseling for shared decision making in addition to annual screening for beneficiaries who meet the eligibility criteria (which is similar to the NLST trial eligibility criteria). Consequently, lung cancer screening without patient cost sharing is now a preventive service benefit for many Americans (CMS, 2015; USPSTF, 2014).

However, many factors need to be considered for broad implementation of lung cancer screening in clinical practice. Massetti said that effective implementation will entail

- Understanding the balance of potential benefits and harms of lung cancer screening;
- Facilitating informed, shared decision making;
- Defining and reaching eligible populations;

---

[2] The USPSTF defined high risk as adults ages 55 to 80 years who have a 30 pack-year smoking history and currently smoke or have quit within the past 15 years (USPSTF, 2014).

[3] Certain private insurance plans (grandfathered plans) are exempt from this requirement (CMS, 2016).

- Determining health system needs, infrastructure requirements, and capacity constraints;
- Coordinating screening efforts with smoking cessation interventions;
- Monitoring outcomes for individual patients and at the population level; and
- Addressing health disparities.

In recognition of the substantial challenges to developing effective lung cancer screening programs in clinical practice, the National Cancer Policy Forum of the National Academies of Sciences, Engineering, and Medicine held a workshop, "Implementation of Lung Cancer Screening" on June 20 and June 21, 2016, in Washington, DC. At the workshop, experts described the current evidence base for lung cancer screening, the current challenges of implementation, and opportunities to overcome them. Workshop discussions also highlighted capacity and access issues; best practices for screening programs; assessment of patient outcomes, quality, and value in lung cancer screening; and research needs that could improve implementation efforts. This proceedings chronicles the presentations and discussions at the workshop. A broad range of views and ideas were presented, and a summary of suggestions for potential actions from individual participants is provided in Box 1. The workshop Statement of Task can be found in Appendix A and the workshop agenda can be found in Appendix B. Speakers' presentations (as PDF and video files) have been archived online.[4]

EVIDENCE BASE FOR LUNG CANCER SCREENING

Prior to the advent of LDCT screening for lung cancer, previous strategies were evaluated, including the use of X-ray imaging. Two trials—the Mayo Lung Project and the Prostate, Lung, Colorectal, and Ovarian Cancer Screening Trial (PLCO)—found that X-ray imaging was ineffective at reducing deaths from lung cancer (Marcus et al., 2000; Oken et al., 2011). "It does not work—that is the bottom line," said Michael LeFevre, professor and director of clinical services at the University of Missouri School of Medicine.

A meta-analysis of LDCT lung cancer screening data conducted by the USPSTF led the group to conclude that "strong evidence shows that

[4] See http://www.nationalacademies.org/hmd/Activities/Disease/NCPF/2016-JUN-20.aspx (accessed August 1, 2016).

BOX 1
Suggestions Made by Individual Workshop Participants to Improve Implementation of Lung Cancer Screening

Ensuring Patient Eligibility and Access to Lung Cancer Screening

- Have clinicians and screening programs confirm that individuals meet eligibility criteria for lung cancer screening in order to maximize benefits and minimize harm from screening. (Aberle, Bach, Black, Mazzone)
- Enhance efforts to reach individuals at high risk for lung cancer and improve access to screening through collaboration among federal, state, and community organizations. (Lathan, Smith, Wood)
- Assist clinicians in identifying patients at high risk for lung cancer by capturing smoking history in electronic medical records. (Lathan, Latimer)
- Centralize the eligibility assessment and the shared decision-making process. (Black)
- Facilitate access to diagnostic and treatment services if patients have positive scans. (Copeland)
- Develop and use patient information materials targeted at difficult-to-reach individuals who are at high risk for lung cancer. (Volk)
- Convey information about lung cancer screening using methods that resonate with different types of learners. (Latimer, Mills, Park)
- Evaluate screening demand versus existing capacity of lung cancer screening programs, imaging equipment, and medical professionals involved in screening and downstream care. (Roth, Smieliauskas)

Improving Shared Decision Making

- Integrate patients' values in the decision-making process for screening and engage family members in the shared decision-making process. (Chambers, Mills)
- Convey information about an individual's risk of lung cancer and other smoking-related diseases to the patient. (Park, Volk)
- Standardize and routinely update decision aids used in shared decision making so they reflect current knowledge about how to express potential benefit, harm, and risk. (Smith)
- Ensure clinicians convey a balanced presentation of potential benefits and harms and avoid fear-based appeals when discussing lung cancer screening with patients. (Volk)

- Designate nurses, decision coaches, or patient navigators who can effectively engage patients in consistent, high-quality shared decision making. (Hoffman, Schneider, Volk)
- In assessing the quality of lung cancer screening programs, do not use the proportion of the eligible population who receive screening, but rather the level of comfort an individual has with their screening decision, based on their values and risks. (Massetti)

Linking Lung Cancer Screening to Smoking Cessation Interventions

- Ensure that access to tobacco cessation services are a required component of the lung cancer screening process. (Lathan)
- Enhance training and technical assistance for smoking cessation within lung cancer screening programs. (Ostroff, Park, Studts)
- Provide consistent smoking cessation messaging to patients who undergo annual lung cancer screening. (Park)
- Engage other relevant clinicians, such respiratory therapists, in low-resource settings to provide needed services. (Stoms)

Minimizing Harms from Lung Cancer Screening

- Assess a patient's comorbidities, life expectancy, ability to undergo further diagnostic evaluations and treatments, and willingness to adhere to annual screening exams when determining eligibility for and appropriateness of screening. (Hoffman)
- Evaluate the performance of Lung-RADS structured reporting and management protocols to detect lung cancers and reduce the risk of unnecessary interventions for false positives and overdiagnosis. (Kazerooni)
- Increase measurement and tracking of health outcomes for individuals who are screened. (Massetti)
- Increase collaboration and guidance between primary care clinicians and radiology and pulmonology clinicians to ensure appropriate screening and referrals for diagnostic procedures and treatment. (Hoffman)

Improving the Quality of Lung Cancer Screening Programs

- Identify the essential components of a lung cancer screening program and leverage successful implementation strategies from other institutions. (Black, Mazzone)
- Consider lung cancer screening as a complex process and recognize that breakdowns in any step could lead to patient harm. (Doria-Rose)
- Develop a set of process and outcomes measures related to smoking cessation for registering lung cancer screening sites. (Ostroff)

continued

BOX 1 Continued

- Clarify the roles and expectations of primary care clinicians in the lung cancer screening process. (Hoffman)
- Develop an imaging atlas that will help radiologists calibrate the interpretation of lung cancer screening images across centers. (Aberle)
- Use computer-aided detection and improve automated structured reporting for lung cancer screening. (Black)
- Monitor the outcomes from lung cancer screening by participating in the CMS-approved ACR Lung Cancer Screening Registry. (Kazerooni)
- Evaluate whether and how quality measurement could be beneficial to improving lung cancer screening implementation. (Bach, Blumenfrucht, Hoffman, LeFevre)

Addressing Research Needs

- Evaluate alternative strategies for identifying individuals at high risk for lung cancer in clinical practice settings. (Tammemägi, Wood)
- Routinely assess capacity needs and strategies to meet these needs to help overcome health disparities in underserved areas. (Smith)
- Enroll diverse, representative populations in clinical trials early by embedding trials within community care settings and leveraging the clinicians and the local medical centers where these individuals will be treated. (Aberle)
- Conduct economic evaluations of lung cancer screening using real-world data from community practices. (Roth)
- Estimate the return on investment of future lung cancer screening clinical trials to prioritize studies and resources. (Roth)
- Conduct more research on how to effectively integrate tobacco cessation programs into lung cancer screening. (Lathan, Ostroff)
- Assess best practices in terms of cost per quit rate and determine treatment implementation strategies needed to establish and maintain cessation in real-world settings. (Ostroff)
- Study communication between patients and clinicians in lung cancer screening programs to minimize breakdowns in the process. (Doria-Rose)

LDCT screening can reduce lung cancer and all-cause mortality. The harms associated with screening must be balanced with the benefits" (USPSTF, 2016a). The meta-analysis included the NLST, the Danish Lung Cancer Screening Trial (DLCST), and the Detection and Screening of Early Lung Cancer by Novel Imaging Technology and Molecular Essays (DANTE) trial in Italy. The NLST trial found that high-risk patients screened with LDCT had a 20 percent reduction in mortality from lung cancer (The National Lung Screening Trial Research Team et al., 2011). The DLCST found no statistically significant effects of LDCT screening on lung cancer mortality, said Peter Bach, director of the Center for Health Policy and Outcomes at Memorial Sloan Kettering Cancer Center. However, subgroup analyses of the DLCST indicated that nonsignficant trends seemed to be in agreement with the NLST (Wille et al., 2016). The DANTE trial had limited statistical power and was not able to assess the effect of LDCT on lung cancer mortality (Infante et al., 2015). LeFevre added that ongoing trials could provide additional information, including the European NELSON (Nederlands-Leuvens Longkanker Screenings Onderzoek) trial (Yousaf-Khan et al., 2015, 2016), which he called "probably the most important [lung cancer screening] trial that is out there right now."

V. Paul Doria-Rose, an epidemiologist in the Division of Cancer Control and Population Sciences at the National Cancer Institute (NCI), noted that the number of cancer deaths prevented by lung cancer screening varies substantially according to level of risk for lung cancer within a population. He added that in the NLST trial, approximately 90 percent of the deaths prevented occurred in the top three quintiles of risk (Kovalchik et al., 2013). Compared to the NLST, the entry criteria for the DLCST were more lenient and included a lower risk population in terms of both age and smoking history, added LeFevre. "The benefits and harms of screening depend on the context in which it occurs including the underlying risk for lung cancer death in the patient populations being screened," he said.

LeFevre said that the reduction in all-cause mortality seen in the meta-analysis was due in part to the poor prognosis associated with a diagnosis of lung cancer: within the control arm of the meta-analysis, approximately one-third of all deaths were attributed to lung cancer. LeFevre added that even though the relative reduction of mortality was not exceptionally large, the absolute risk of lung cancer was so high among this population that the small relative reduction was important.

The NLST data showed that over the 6.5 years, there were 18 deaths from lung cancer for every 1,000 high-risk individuals screened with LDCT

(NCI, 2016b). LeFevre added that compared to X-ray imaging, 3 annual screenings with LDCT averted 3 lung cancer–related deaths for every 1,000 high-risk individuals screened. This is comparable to the number of deaths averted with screening mammography in women ages 50 to 59, according to LeFevre. Douglas Wood, professor and chief of cardiothoracic surgery at the University of Washington, added that lung cancer screening is relatively efficient, with the number needed to screen[5] (320 over 6.5 years in the NLST) lower than that for other cancer screenings (mammography for women who are ages 60-69 = 377 over 11 to 20 years; colonoscopy = 871 over 12 years) (The National Lung Screening Trial Research Team, 2011; Nelson et al., 2009; Schoen et al., 2012).

However, lung cancer screening also has the potential for harm, said LeFevre, including a high false-positive rate, overdiagnosis,[6] and complications associated from evaluating and treating suspected lung cancers found on screening, as well as complications from evaluating and treating incidental findings. For example, in the NLST, the rate of positive results in the LDCT arm was 24.2 percent, but approximately 96 percent of these positive results were false positives (The National Lung Screening Trial Research Team, 2011). Although a high percentage of these false positives were resolved with subsequent imaging, over the course of the trial, 25 out of every 1,000 individuals screened had a false alarm that led to an invasive procedure, such as a bronchoscopy, biopsy, or surgery; 3 out of every 1,000 people screened had a major complication from invasive procedures (NCI, 2016b). Of 17,053 positive screening results during the entire course of the trial, there were 61 complications and 6 deaths following a diagnostic procedure (or a rate of approximately 1 in 5,000 people screened who did not have lung cancer but died following a diagnostic procedure) (USPSTF, 2014). This is in contrast to 15-20 people out of every 5,000 high-risk individuals screened who would have a lung cancer death averted by the screening, LeFevre said. He added that "it was the USPSTF judgment that the number of deaths averted [from lung cancer screening] was great enough to justify" the potential complications from screening. "But that does not mean that screening is harmless," LeFevre said.

Doria-Rose added that the false-positive rate varies considerably

---

[5] The number needed to screen is the number of people who need to be screened to prevent one bad outcome (lung cancer–related death).

[6] Overdiagnosis occurs "when a condition is diagnosed that would otherwise not go on to cause symptoms or death" (Welch and Black, 2010, p. 605).

according to the experience of the radiologist interpreting the LDCT scan. Even within the NLST, in which radiologists were required to have experience with LDCT lung scans and undergo additional training, one study found the false-positive rate varied between 4 and 69 percent for radiologists who interpreted the highest volume of scans (i.e., read at least 100 screening exams over the course of the trial) (Pinsky et al., 2013). "Even in the much more controlled environment of the NLST, there was considerable variation in the performance of the radiologists. We will see how that translates into the community," Doria-Rose said.

The complication rate for diagnostic procedures is greater among patients with concurrent illnesses (comorbidities), such as heart disease and chronic obstructive pulmonary disorder (COPD), which are common in individuals who smoke, said Bach. "The tradeoff . . . of increasing comorbidity is excess mortality or morbidity from complications, probably including complications from responses to false positives. These are all drags on the benefit of screening," Bach said. "This particular intervention is a real tightrope walk on the evidence: if you cannot get all of the efficacy and the low rates of harm we saw in the NLST, then it looks like a very unappealing thing for a long list of patients," he added. Doria-Rose noted that one study found that individuals who had two or more respiratory comorbidities saw no benefit of screening (Kovalchik et al., 2013). "As you translate [LDCT screening] into the community where we may be seeing more people with more comorbid conditions, we may see a different efficacy of screening," he said. On average the NLST participants were younger, had higher educational status, and had fewer comorbidities than the general screening-eligible population (The National Lung Screening Trial Research Team, 2010; Pinsky et al., 2014).

The complication rate also can vary by institution and experience of the clinician performing the diagnostic and/or treatment procedures, and is also likely to be higher outside the academic settings that participated in the NLST, Doria-Rose said. For example, a population-based estimate of the risk of complications from lung nodule biopsies found that the pneumothorax (or a collapsed lung) complication rate from needle biopsies occurred in approximately 15 percent of lung biopsies, but this rate varied substantially (from 0 to 50 percent) among the hospitals surveyed; although the rate of hemorrhage from needle biopsies was low (1 percent), it varied from 0 to 6 percent (Wiener et al., 2011). Other studies have found that the mortality linked to a lobectomy (surgical removal of a lobe of the lung) ranged from 3 to 6 percent in community hospitals, while the NLST reported a mortality rate of approximately 1 percent for that procedure (Bach et al., 2001; The National Lung Screening Trial Research Team et al., 2011; Silvestri et al., 1998). Denise Aberle, vice chair of radiology and professor at the University of California School of Medicine, agreed that the NLST surgical mortality was unusually low and said that it was probably due to the dedicated subspecialty thoracic surgeons who conducted the surgeries. Participating facilities in the NLST tended to be NCI-designated cancer centers with a lot of expertise, Bach added. Doria-Rose explained that "there is variability in how lung cancer screening is going to perform in different settings due both to differences in the patient populations that are being screened as well as the performance of providers who are delivering and interpreting the screening test, and then downstream, performing diagnostic testing and treating cancers that are diagnosed. Consequently, what we observe in real-world settings with respect to risk–benefit ratio may be different from what was seen in the NLST."

Robert Smith, vice president of cancer screening at the American Cancer Society (ACS), acknowledged the concern that the high-quality care provided in the NLST trial may not always be replicable in community settings. But he noted that ACS has convened a National Lung Cancer Screening Roundtable, composed of more than 70 organizations, to address the challenges of implementing high-quality screening in the community setting. He added that we are "not going to be able to achieve high-quality lung cancer screening if we do not start doing it and start learning from our experiences."

Annual screening with LDCT also results in exposure to radiation, which has the potential for harm, including the development of cancer. LeFevre said the radiation dose in LDCT is much lower than the dose used for diagnostic scans and is comparable to mammography. However, he noted the impact of radiation is cumulative, so the earlier screening begins, the more likely the radiation could be harmful over time. Furthermore, if LDCT scans indicate the need for additional follow-up, diagnostic imaging will increase the risk of radiation harms.

Another harm linked to lung cancer screening is overdiagnosis because some people will be treated for lung cancers that would not have caused them harm. An analysis of NLST data found that the probability of a lung cancer being overdiagnosed is 18.5 percent; for every lung cancer death averted by the screening, 1.38 lung cancers are overdiagnosed (Patz et al., 2014). But LeFevre added that he thought these estimates of overdiagnosis were probably high, due to the short length of follow-up time (4 to 5 years following screening), which could have underestimated the number of cancers in the X-ray screening group.

In addition, the high likelihood that individuals will experience false-positive screening results prompted concern that the screening might cause psychological harm. However, LeFevre reported that analyses reviewed by the USPSTF did not find that screening has resulted in long-term psychological distress or anxiety, although assessment has been limited (USPSTF, 2014).

Approximately 8 percent of those screened in the NLST had clinically significant incidental findings unrelated to lung cancer (e.g., cardiac abnormalities, COPD, aneurysms, or masses in other tissues), said LeFevre. Barnet Kramer, director of the NCI Division of Cancer Prevention, added that many incidental findings have unknown significance. Some patients benefit from their detection, Kramer said. More often, they do not benefit. Sometimes a finding is unlikely to cause problems in the future. Other times, the diagnostic procedure itself is harmful, including when a finding is difficult to biopsy and results indicate that further treatment is not needed. For example, the LDCT scans used in lung cancer screening can detect small, slow-growing kidney tumors that are not likely to be harmful but are difficult to access. Ella Kazerooni, professor of radiology at the University of Michigan, noted that the American College of Radiology (ACR) has management guidelines for incidental findings of the abdomen and thyroid gland, and is currently developing management guidelines for incidental findings in the chest.

Wood noted that "in preventive services, harm presents itself in two forms: one is the unintended consequences of evaluation and treatment. But there is also the harm that comes from denying preventive services from those who may benefit." He added "The NLST creates an important foundation for our guidelines and what we do, but it is only a foundation for them. We do have to consider other risk factors, as well as how we deliver lung cancer screening responsibly and minimize risk not just by limiting access [only to high-risk patients], but also by improving management of the patients that are screened."

Several participants pointed out that risk for harms from lung cancer screening could potentially be minimized with appropriate management of screening results and improved surgical techniques. Kazerooni indicated that Lung-RADS is expected to reduce the positive screen rate from approximately 1 in 10 to 1 in 25 (Pinsky et al., 2015), thereby reducing follow-up testing and radiation exposure, as well as invasive procedures, overdiagnosis, and patient anxiety. "Just because we find something does not mean we have to do something about it. . . . Many of these [findings] can be observed for prolonged and potentially indefinite periods of time," Wood said. He often has conversations with patients who have had lung cancer screening to describe why a detected lung nodule that is likely to be harmless does not have to be removed. "This is what we should be doing and is part of diminishing the unintended harms of lung cancer screening," Wood said. The harms from surgery may also be lessened by recent advances in surgical technique, such as minimally invasive thoracoscopic surgery to remove lung tissue, pointed out Aberle (Iñiguez et al., 2016). "As thoracoscopic resection becomes the norm, which it is for most lobectomies already, the 3 to 5 percent mortality rate will [decrease]," she said.

ELIGIBILITY, CLINICAL PRACTICE GUIDELINES, AND MODELING

Some workshop participants provided a comparison of the current recommendations for screening from various clinical practice guidelines, the USPSTF, and an overview of the current eligibility requirements for lung cancer screening under the CMS national coverage decision; the potential role of risk modeling to refine eligibility; and concerns about guideline adherence in clinical practice. Table 1 provides an overview of the current eligibility criteria for lung cancer screening.

TABLE 1 Overview of the Current Eligibility Criteria for LDCT Lung Cancer Screening

Organizations	Eligibility Criteria
U.S. Preventive Services Task Force (USPSTF)	The USPSTF recommends annual screening for lung cancer with low-dose computed tomography in adults ages 55 to 80 years who have a 30 pack-year smoking history and currently smoke or have quit within the past 15 years. Screening should be discontinued once a person has not smoked for 15 years or develops a health problem that substantially limits life expectancy or the ability or willingness to have curative lung surgery.

TABLE 1 Continued

Organizations	Eligibility Criteria
Centers for Medicare & Medicaid Services National Coverage Determination on Lung Cancer Screening	People ages 55 to 77 with at least a 30 pack-year smoking history and who currently smoke or have quit within the past 15 years. Medicare coverage includes a visit for counseling and shared decision making on the potential benefits and risks of lung cancer screening. The National Coverage Determination also includes required data collection and specific coverage eligibility criteria for radiologists and radiology imaging centers, consistent with the National Lung Screening Trial (NLST) protocol, USPSTF recommendation, and multisociety, multidisciplinary, stakeholder evidence-based guidelines.
Clinical Practice Guidelines from ACCP, ACS, ALA, ASCO, ATS, GOLF, IASLC, IFCT	Follow the NLST eligibility criteria. People ages 55 to 74 with at least a 30 pack-year smoking history and who currently or formerly smoke.
National Comprehensive Cancer Network	People ages 55 to 74 with at least a 30 pack-year smoking history and who currently smoke or have quit within the past 15 years. People ages 50 and older with at least a 20 pack-year smoking history and an additional risk factor for lung cancer. Additional risk factors include occupational or environmental exposures, a personal or family history of cancer, and additional lung diseases, such as COPD and pulmonary fibrosis, but not second-hand smoking. The same criteria are recommended by the American Academy of Thoracic Surgeons.
American Academy of Family Physicians	The evidence is insufficient to recommend for or against screening for lung cancer with LDCT.

NOTE: ACCP = American College of Chest Physicians; ACS = American Cancer Society; ALA = American Lung Association; ASCO = American Society of Clinical Oncology; ATS = American Thoracic Society; GOLF = Groupe d'Oncologie de Langue Française; IASLC = International Association for the Study of Lung Cancer; IFCT = French Cooperative Thoracic Intergroup; LDCT = low-dose computed tomography.
SOURCES: Adapted from Bach, Chin, LeFevre, and Wood presentations, June 20, 2016; Borgmeyer, 2014; CMS, 2015; Wood et al., 2012.

All recommendations for lung cancer screening specify that individuals should be asymptomatic at the time of screening. But there was some discussion about the definition of asymptomatic for individuals at high risk of developing lung cancer. Joanna Stoms, cancer plan manager at the Pennsylvania Department of Health, noted that a patient with a 30 pack-year history of smoking often presents with some symptoms of COPD, such as shortness of breath or persistent cough, that could also mimic signs of lung cancer. Richard Hoffman, professor of internal medicine and director of the division of general internal medicine at the University of Iowa Carver College of Medicine, also said many patients who are eligible for lung cancer screening may have a cough, shortness of breath, or wheezing. Other signs and symptoms that would suggest they are ineligible for lung cancer screening (but instead need diagnostic evaluation) would include coughing up blood, unexplained weight loss, fever, night sweats, and other symptoms beyond just a cough and difficulty breathing, Hoffman added. Kazerooni agreed that it can be challenging to set criteria for assessing whether an individual who smokes is asymptomatic or not. "It is an enriched sample. There are a lot of people who may be at risk for lung cancer who have these indolent symptoms that are different than just the usual smoker's cough or smoker's sputum product that may be coming out for screenings. But how do you actually codify what is normal for a smoker?" Kazerooni asked. Criteria could include questions to assess how much a person coughs, how much sputum is produced, or how those have changed over time. However, individuals may have difficulty assessing whether their symptoms are normal for them. That difficulty may explain, in part, the higher rate of positive screens than was expected with lung cancer screening, she said.

There has been some disagreement about identifying the appropriate high-risk population for lung cancer screening, several workshop participants noted. In Figure 1, Bach illustrated that a majority of clinical practice guidelines have eligibility criteria that are consistent with the NLST in terms of pack-year smoking history[7] and age. However, the USPSTF, the National Comprehensive Cancer Network (NCCN), the CMS national coverage determination, and others have expanded eligibility requirements for lung cancer screening beyond the NLST criteria.

[7] A pack-year is "a way to measure the amount a person has smoked over a long period of time. It is calculated by multiplying the number of packs of cigarettes smoked per day by the number of years the person has smoked. For example, 1 pack-year is equal to smoking 1 pack per day for 1 year, or 2 packs per day for half a year, and so on" (NCI, 2016a).

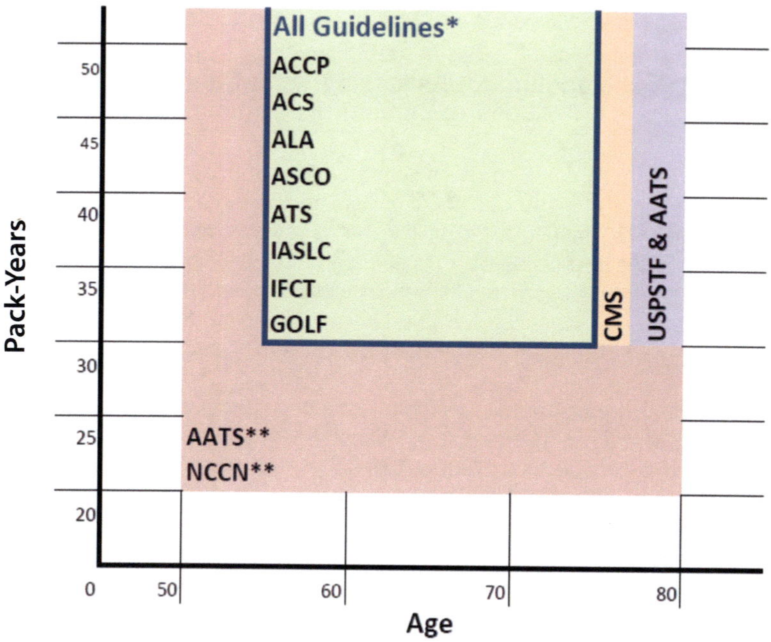

FIGURE 1 Age and smoking pack-year history eligibility criteria for lung cancer screening from different organizations.

NOTES: AATS = American Association for Thoracic Surgery; ACCP = American College of Chest Physicians; ACS = American Cancer Society; ALA = American Lung Association; ASCO = American Society of Clinical Oncology; ATS = American Thoracic Society; CMS = Centers for Medicare & Medicaid Services; GOLF = Groupe d'Oncologie de Langue Française; IASLC = International Association for the Study of Lung Cancer; IFCT = French Cooperative Thoracic Intergroup; LDCT = low-dose computed tomography; NCCN = National Comprehensive Cancer Network; USPSTF = U.S. Preventive Services Task Force.

* American Academy of Family Physicians does not recommend LDCT screening for any populations.

** With an additional risk factor.

SOURCE: Bach presentation, June 20, 2016.

Some research has focused on the development of risk modeling with the intent of improving the selection of individuals for lung cancer screening (see Box 2). LeFevre noted that the USPSTF used modeling to estimate the effects of changing eligibility requirements for lung cancer screening, including expanding screening eligibility up to age 80, which led to the USPSTF recommendation (USPSTF, 2013). Joseph Chin, deputy director of the CMS Coverage and Analysis Group, noted that CMS took into

BOX 2
Risk Modeling for Assessing Lung Cancer Risk and Selecting Screening Participants

Douglas Wood, professor and chief of the Division of Cardiothoracic Surgery at the University of Washington, noted that National Lung Screening Trial (NLST) eligibility criteria reaches approximately 27 percent of the population who will actually develop lung cancer (Pinsky and Berg, 2012). Several workshop participants described current efforts to improve risk modeling for lung cancer screening. Martin Tammemägi, professor of epidemiology at Brock University and senior scientist in prevention and cancer control at Cancer Care Ontario, said there are currently 20 risk-prediction models for lung cancer screening, but most are not practical for population-based screening because they require blood or genetic tests,[a] require extensive medical record data, or are limited to specific populations. Of the models relevant to population-based lung cancer screening, there are a few that apply specifically to individuals who smoke, Tammemägi reported (Bach et al., 2003; Hoggart et al., 2012; Katki et al., 2016; Tammemägi et al. 2013; Wilson and Weissfeld, 2015). He said risk prediction modeling is better at selecting individuals for lung cancer screening than the NLST-like trial eligibility criteria because it can better predict who is at highest risk for developing lung cancer. He noted that the NLST-like criteria tie together smoking duration and intensity (using pack-years), but they do not really truly travel together in a 1 to 1 relationship with risk for lung cancer (Peto, 2012). Another advantage that modeling has over the NLST criteria is that it is more granular when assessing individual risks and includes additional predictors, such as race and ethnicity, in its risk estimation. Although lung cancer risk varies by race and ethnicity, Tammemägi said that the NLST criteria do not incorporate these differences, which can potentially lead to health disparities (Fiscella et al., 2015). Furthermore, risk modeling can include nonlinear relationships as well as additional predictors to improve predictive accuracy.

He described the risk model developed from the Prostate, Lung, Colorectal, and Ovarian Cancer (PLCO) control arm trial data in detail.

account the modeling data from the USPSTF to inform its coverage decision on lung cancer screening, because the Medicare population includes a sizable portion of people over age 74, for whom there are no NLST data.

By expanding the age limit for screening to 80 years, the USPSTF recommendation assumes that the benefits outweigh the harms in this older

The risk model, $PLCO_{m2012}$, was externally validated using the German cohort data from the European Prospective Investigation into Cancer and Nutrition study (Li et al., 2015). Using a risk threshold of 1.5 percent, the $PLCO_{m2012}$ risk model estimated that the number needed to screen to avert one lung cancer death was 255, compared to NLST, which found the number needed to screen was 320 (Tammemägi et al., 2014b).

With the PLCO intervention trial arm data, compared with the USPSTF criteria, the $PLCO_{m2012}$ model was associated with improved sensitivity, specificity, and positive predictive values (Tammemägi et al., 2013, 2014b). Comparison of the two criteria indicated that the PLCO model would screen approximately 9 percent fewer people while identifying about 12 percent more lung cancers.

"Clearly using a reasonable model risk threshold would be much more efficient than using the NLST criteria or the USPSTF criteria for selecting screenees," Tammemägi said. Another advantage of using a risk prediction model such as the PLCO model is that one can enhance and improve it by including additional predictors, such as screening results, he added. If a person's risk borders on the threshold for screening and his/her last screening result was positive, for example, risk increases. But if it was negative, risk can drop below the threshold, so he/she would not need to be screened the following year, he said. Risk based on an earlier version of the PLCO model was used to recruit individuals for screening in the Pan-Canadian Early Detection Lung Cancer study, and was found to identify a relatively high proportion of individuals with lung cancer, according to Tammemägi. The $PLCO_{m2012}$ model risk criteria of greater than 2 percent is also being used to determine entry for Cancer Care Ontario's High-Risk Lung Cancer Screening Pilot Studies. He said the main hurdle for prediction modeling is acceptance and incorporation into lung cancer screening guidelines and programs.

[a] However, Tammemägi suggested that biomarkers could potentially improve the risk prediction models for lung cancer screening, such as the blood level of the serum pro-surfactant protein B, which might be an indicator of lung cancer (Sin et al., 2013). Tammemägi and his colleagues are currently evaluating whether a panel of 10 biomarkers can improve lung cancer prediction modeling.

population, but Bach questioned whether this is assumption is appropriate. Life expectancy falls as people age, so for each lung cancer death averted in an older population, the gain earned is less than it is for a younger person. Bach added that the risk of surgical mortality rises with age, as does the false-positive rate of lung cancer screening. "As you get older in age, you have less life expectancy, are more likely to have a false-positive screen, and are more likely to have harm from screening," Bach said.

Bach noted that some guidelines and institutions are expanding the eligibility criteria for lung cancer screening based on additional lung cancer risk factors beyond pack-years and age, such as occupational and environmental exposure history, family history, and the presence of other lung diseases, such as COPD. However, Bach expressed concern with this approach, noting, "I do not think we can say that a radon-induced cancer is the same as a tobacco-induced cancer, so just plugging something into a model and showing that somebody has the same overall risk does not necessarily translate to the same overall benefit. We are probably safest within the confines of the types of people who have been studied."

Bach also expressed concern about the use of surrogate endpoints in the assessment of lung cancer screening interventions and their inclusion in risk modeling. Bach noted that there are two main surrogate endpoints that are used in lung cancer screening prediction models: survival of those who are diagnosed with cancer through screening (with the assumption that survival is equivalent to 1 – mortality) or the proportion of stage I lung cancers identified, with the assumption that localized detection of lung cancer improves survival. However, the use of survival as an endpoint is susceptible to lead time and length time biases, in part because survival only accounts for patients with cancer in the denominator, whereas the mortality calculation includes all patients who underwent lung cancer screening. While screening could potentially extend survival by identifying cancers before symptoms appear, this earlier identification may have no impact on a clinical outcome, such as mortality.

Bach added that investigators from the International-Early Lung Cancer Action Program (I-ELCAP)—a clinical trial that screened asymptomatic individuals at risk for lung cancer using LDCT—estimated that the 10-year lung cancer–specific survival rate for individuals diagnosed with stage I cancer was 88 percent. Trial investigators concluded that LDCT screening could prevent 80 percent of deaths from lung cancer (The International Early Lung Cancer Action Program Investigators, 2006).

Bach and Wood noted that this estimate was much greater than the 20 percent mortality reduction seen with NLST. To evaluate whether survival or stage I diagnosis of lung cancer could potentially be used as surrogates in the setting of lung cancer, Bach analyzed NLST data from each participating site to see if there was a correlation between mortality and these potential surrogates. Bach found that stage I lung cancer detection and

4-year lung cancer–specific survival were not predictive of mortality using NLST data, nor were they predictive when he used data from the Danish Lung Cancer Screening Trial (DLCST). Both Chin and Bach stressed that the lack of valid surrogates may be due, in part, to the substantial variation in an individual's risk for lung cancer, based on factors such as age, sex, smoking history, and occupational exposure to asbestos (Bach and Gould, 2012) (see Table 2).

Wood noted that the NLST was a clinical trial, and eligibility criteria for enrollment in the trial were never meant to define the extent of "high risk" or be the basis of public policy. He added that the NCCN clinical practice guideline on lung cancer screening was developed by a group of people with a wide range of expertise and uses a combination of evidence and expert consensus to fill in the gaps where evidence does not exist. Recognizing that it is unlikely that another randomized trial of lung cancer screening would be undertaken to assess the effect of other lung cancer risk factors, the NCCN extrapolated from other studies and models, Wood reported. One pooled analysis, for example, found that lung cancer risk was 2.44 times higher in those with emphysema (Brenner et al., 2012). Another analysis compared results for high-risk individuals meeting NLST criteria with the expanded high-risk group identified by the NCCN criteria (ages 50 to 55 with a 20 pack-year smoking history and an additional risk factor) (McKee et al., 2015). Wood said this analysis found that the expanded risk category was substantially similar to the NLST group in terms of positive screening results and lung cancer diagnoses. Andrea Borondy Kitts, a patient advocate, noted that these results are being updated, and although they are not published yet, they also indicate equal incidence of lung cancer in patients who are screened either by the NLST or NCCN eligibility criteria.

Wood added that NCCN guidelines on lung cancer screening provide specific algorithms for managing solid or non-solid nodules detected, and lists the potential risks and benefits for each option that can help inform a shared decision-making conversation with patients. "We can use management algorithms to minimize false positives and the consequences of false positives," he said.

Wood added that using NLST criteria, approximately 9 million people would be eligible for lung cancer screening, and 12,250 annual deaths from lung cancer could potentially be averted (Ma et al., 2013). If NCCN eligibility criteria were applied, Wood said that another 2 million people would be eligible for screening and potentially 3,000 additional annual deaths from lung cancer could be averted (Ma et al., 2013; McKee et al., 2015).

TABLE 2 Projected Likelihood Over 6 Years of Lung Cancer Death with or Without Screening per 1,000 Persons Screened[a]

Participant	Risk Factors	Deaths from Lung Cancer (Without Screening) per 1,000 Persons, *n*
"Typical" participant in the NSLT	62-year-old male current 1.5-PPD smoker for 35 years	19.50
Minimum eligible participant in the NLST	55-year-old female former 1-PPD smoker for 30 years who just quit	4.00
High-risk participant in the NLST	70-year-old current 2-PPD smoker for 55 years	60.90
Minimum eligible participant by NCCN guidelines	50-year-old male former smoker 1-PPD smoker for 20 years who quit 10 years ago with an occupational asbestos exposure history	1.60
Low-risk eligible participant for Sequoia Hospital lung screening program	40-year-old female former 1-PPD smoker for 10 years who quit 15 years ago	0.10

NOTE: NCCN = National Comprehensive Cancer Network; NLST = National Lung Screening Trial; PPD = packs per day.

[a] Assuming the program includes 3 years of annual screening.

Representativeness of the NLST Population

Several workshop participants noted there is some concern about the representativeness of the NLST population, the results of which have largely set the recommendations for lung cancer screening implementation in clinical practice. Bach said that compared to the general population of tobacco users surveyed by the U.S. Census Bureau's Tobacco Use Supplement, those who participated in the NLST were substantially younger, had higher educational status, and were more likely to be former smokers (The

Deaths from Lung Cancer (with Screening) per 1,000 Persons, *n*	Lung Cancer Deaths Averted per 1,000 Persons, *n*	Persons Needed to Be Screened Annually for 3 Years to Prevent 1 Death from Lung Cancer Over 6 Years, *n*
15.60	3.90	256
3.20	0.80	1,236
48.70	12.20	82
1.30	0.30	3,180
0.08	0.02	35,186

SOURCES: Bach presentation, June 20, 2016; From *Annals of Internal Medicine*, Bach, Peter B.; Gould, Michael K., When the Average Applies to No One: Personalized Decision Making About Potential Benefits of Lung Cancer Screening, 157, 8, 571-573.

National Lung Screening Trial Research Team et al., 2010). Bach said that higher educational attainment is linked to higher screening adherence rates, which will be key to the efficacy of lung cancer screening. Furthermore, Bach noted that none of the NLST participants were older than age 74 years at trial entry, so there are no data on the efficacy of lung cancer screening beyond this age, nor is there information on screening for longer durations than in the NLST trial, which included three annual screens and 6.5 years of follow-up.

Christopher Lathan, assistant professor of medicine at Harvard Medical School and director of the Cancer Care Equity Program at the Dana-Farber Cancer Institute, said that African Americans and people of lower socioeconomic status who are not college educated have the highest risk of developing and dying from lung cancer, yet these populations were underrepresented in the NLST (Albano et al., 2007; The National Lung Screening Trial Research Team, 2010). A subgroup analysis of NLST found that lung cancer screening decreased mortality in all groups, but especially among African Americans, who were on average younger, less educated, and had more comorbidities than the general NLST population (Tanner et al., 2015). He added that there are many calls to limit lung cancer screening to the findings of the NLST, "but we have not really increased access to people who probably need it the most," such as African Americans who smoke, Lathan noted. Wood agreed and suggested that the NCCN eligibility expansion could help address current disparities in lung cancer mortality. Citing the ACS 2015 goal to eliminate disparities in cancer burden in different segments of the U.S. population, Wood said that expanding access to lung cancer screening "is especially relevant because disparities in health care disproportionately affect patients at risk for lung cancer."

Adherence to Clinical Practice Guidelines

Several workshop participants expressed concern that clinicians and institutions would not adhere to lung cancer screening guidelines. Jane Kim, acting chief consultant for preventive medicine at the Department of Veterans Affairs (VA), noted that "you can tell providers what the eligibility criteria are, but they may not remember exactly or apply them consistently." Doria-Rose added, "Documentation of eligibility can be difficult. Consequently, screening is occurring outside of eligibility guidelines." Bach said that "We have to be cautious because the march into other populations is upon us. There are facilities out there happy to screen people outside of the guidelines." In an analysis, Bach found that approximately 19 percent of the Lung Cancer Alliance's (LCA's) trusted screening sites followed the NLST criteria and 13 percent followed the USPSTF criteria (Ong, 2014). Bach reported that there is also variability in eligibility requirements applied within large academic cancer centers, with NCCN member institutions often using different eligibility criteria (see Figure 2).

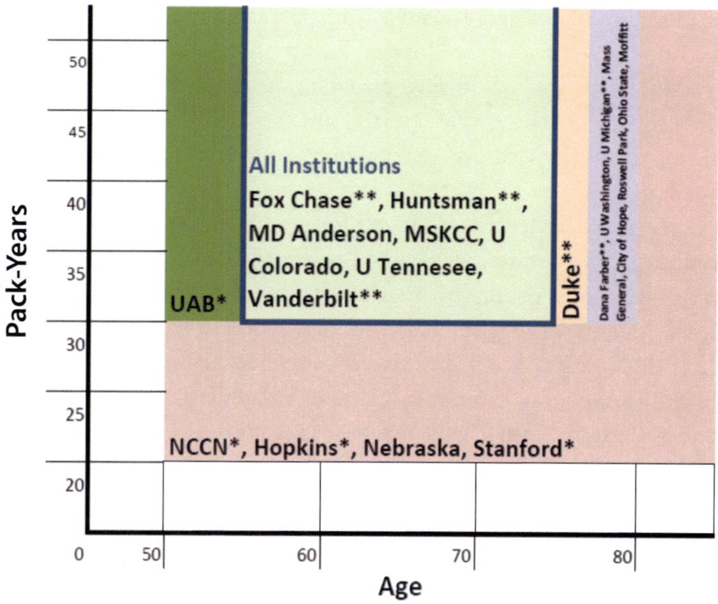

FIGURE 2 Variability in lung cancer screening among different institutions.
NOTES: MSKCC = Memorial Sloan Kettering Cancer Center; NCCN = National Comprehensive Cancer Network; UAB = The University of Alabama at Birmingham.
* With an additional risk factor.
** Technically does not state their own recommendations. Moffitt's website states that an ineligible individual with a physician's referral may be screened.
SOURCE: Bach presentation, June 20, 2016.

INSURANCE COVERAGE OF LUNG CANCER SCREENING

Workshop participants also discussed insurance coverage of lung cancer screening, including issues with private insurance, Medicaid coverage, as well as the CMS Medicare national coverage determination for lung cancer screening.

Although the ACA requires many private insurers to cover lung cancer screening without coinsurance if the USPSTF eligibility requirements are met, several workshop participants said that insurance coverage can still limit access. For example, although the initial LDCT screening may not require coinsurance (or patient cost sharing), if individuals have findings that require additional diagnostic follow-up, people may have out-of-pocket costs for additional imaging or biopsies, Kazerooni noted.

In addition, individuals insured through state Medicaid programs have variable access to preventive care services, and there may be challenges with eligible individuals in Medicaid seeking preventive care, said Otis Brawley, chief medical officer at the ACS. More than half of states have expanded Medicaid coverage under the ACA, and for individuals enrolled under the Medicaid expansion, states are required to cover USPSTF-recommended prevention services without cost sharing. However, for adults enrolled in traditional Medicaid programs, states are not required to cover USPSTF-recommended services, but can receive enhanced federal matching funds if they cover these services without cost sharing (Gates et al., 2014). Brawley added that patients with Medicaid insurance may not seek care when asymptomatic, even if they are eligible for lung cancer screening without out-of-pocket costs.

CMS National Coverage Determination on Lung Cancer Screening

Chin said a sizable proportion of individuals at high risk for lung cancer are insured through the Medicare program because it covers people ages 65 and older, and on average, lung cancer is diagnosed when patients are 70 years old (NCI, 2016c). In light of this, CMS convened the Medicare Evidence Development and Coverage Advisory Committee (MEDCAC) to review the evidence on lung cancer screening. The MEDCAC concluded that there was low confidence that there was adequate evidence of the benefits of lung cancer screening outweighing the harms in the Medicare population (Crawford, 2014). The MEDCAC noted significant evidence gaps in the effects of lung cancer screening for people in the Medicare population who do not meet the eligibility criteria used in the clinical trial, and concern about the potential for overdiagnosis, higher false-positive rates, more diagnostic evaluations of nodules, and higher mortality rates in older adults. Given these concerns, the MEDCAC convened several meetings with various stakeholders, including professional societies and patient advocates. "We wanted to get a sense of how we could implement a high-quality screening program in the Medicare population to detect lung cancer," Chin said. The end result was a national coverage decision for Medicare beneficiaries up to age 77 who are asymptomatic and have at least a 30 pack-year smoking history and are current smokers or have quit smoking within the past 15 years.

CMS specified a number of requirements for coverage: "We did not feel comfortable just saying that we would cover it straight out without any other criteria. Instead we have a number of specific criteria for coverage, probably more than for our typical coverage decisions," Chin noted. For example, Medicare patients need to participate in a counseling and shared decision-making visit with their clinician prior to lung cancer screening. In addition, patients who are screened will have the results of the screening entered into a registry to track outcomes, said Chin.

The coverage decision also defined criteria that radiologists must meet to interpret LDCT images for lung cancer screening. Imaging facilities also had to meet certain standards, including imaging within a low-dose range, offering smoking cessation interventions for current smokers, and collection and submission of data to a CMS-approved registry for every LDCT scan performed. "We want to track this and look at real-world registry data and ultimately link it to our administrative claims data to look at some outcomes and how this actually plays out over time," Chin said. "Based on the data collected, we want to try to refine the criteria that we use and also refine the shared decision-making requirements," he said. "As we get more real-world data perhaps we will have a better sense as to what the criteria for screening should be, especially in the older age ranges."

CMS coverage of lung cancer screening also has several requirements of clinicians to ensure that the eligible population is being screened and that patients are aware of the potential benefits and risks of that screening. These requirements are

- To determine if patient eligibility requirements for screening are met, including age, absence of signs or symptoms of lung cancer, and appropriate smoking history;
- To engage in shared decision making, including the use of one or more decision aids that has information on the potential benefits and harms of screening, follow-up diagnostic testing, overdiagnosis, false-positive rates, and total radiation exposure;
- To provide counseling on the importance of adhering to annual lung cancer LDCT screening, the impact of comorbidities, and ability or willingness to undergo diagnosis and treatment; and
- To provide counseling on the importance of continuing to avoid smoking if a former smoker, or the importance of smoking cessation if a current smoker and, if appropriate, to provide information about tobacco cessation interventions.

CMS established two specific codes for lung cancer screening—one for the shared decision-making visit and one for the LDCT imaging—so that clinicians can be reimbursed for providing the counseling visit, even if the patient ultimately declines to undergo the scanning. Chin noted that the main purpose of the initial required visit is to consider specific patient characteristics, such as comorbidities or ability to undergo screening, diagnostic procedures, and treatment, as well as to enable patients and clinicians to discuss issues such as overdiagnosis, false-positive rates, and commitment to annual screening.

After a patient visit for counseling and shared decision making, clinicians can provide an order for screening if appropriate. However, preliminary data collected by CMS suggest that the shared decision making is not occurring as frequently as it should. Thus far, the number of reported shared decision-making visits is approximately 1,000, but nearly 9,000 scans have been performed, Chin reported. "We would expect more of a one-to-one type of ratio because we made it a requirement to have the shared decision-making visit before starting screening," he noted, but added that the data are not yet complete. CMS will be evaluating this situation to make sure there is better alignment counseling and scan claims. LeFevre suggested that the lower-than-expected claims might be due to office personnel not realizing they can bill CMS for the counseling visit. "I have referred several people to our lung cancer screening program and counseled all of them. I doubt that any one of them was picked up by our billing office. I do not find the discrepancy between claims and screens shocking from where I live and work," he said.

SHARED DECISION MAKING

Several workshop speakers discussed Medicare's requirement for shared decision making, including the definition of the term, why it is important, who should provide it, and what tools and training can facilitate its use. Robert Volk, professor at the University of Texas MD Anderson Cancer Center, defined shared decision making:

> Shared decision making is a collaborative process that allows patients and their providers to make health care decisions together. It takes into account the best clinical evidence available, as well as the patient's values and preferences. Shared decision making is not a goal. The goal is better health decisions to achieve outcomes that matter most to the patient. And shared decision making is a way to reach that goal. A proven process to incorporate the patient's

> voice in health care decisions, shared decision making is the pinnacle of patient-centered care. (Healthwise, 2016)

"Often there is a misconception about shared decision making—that it somehow pulls the clinician out of the decision-making process. That is not the case at all. Shared decision making very much relies on the provider's expert knowledge," Volk stressed. Shonta Chambers, executive vice president of Health Equity Initiatives and Programs for the Patient Advocate Foundation, highlighted the need for patient values to influence decision making. "We focus so much on what is the matter *with* the patient that we do not focus so much on what matters *to* the patient," she said. Ide Mills, a patient advocate and lung cancer survivor, suggested that family members be incorporated into the shared decision-making process so that patients can discuss the screening with people who they trust, know their values, and care about their welfare.

Bach noted that all guidelines for lung cancer screening recommend shared decision making. "They all say at some level, 'we have the data but you need to approach people and propose screening, not mandate it.'" Bach added that shared decision making is important because the potential risks and benefits of lung cancer screening are highly variable and dependent on a patient's individual risk of developing lung cancer. Some people eligible for lung cancer screening may be younger and have a shorter smoking history, and thus their probability of benefiting from screening is reduced.

Peter Mazzone, director of the Lung Cancer Screening Program at the Cleveland Clinic, added that he has found that some eligible patients opt out of lung cancer screening after undergoing shared decision making because they would not accept treatment, even if they were found to have a localized cancer. "Some patients have a lot of comorbidities and they make very reasonable choices that we as physicians struggle to make," he said. "It is a small but real and significant number of patients who opt out for this reason."

Jamie Studts, associate professor at the University of Kentucky College of Medicine and director of behavioral and community-based research at the Markey Cancer Center, noted that shared decision making is important because long-term adherence and engagement with screening programs is needed to reduce lung cancer mortality: "There is no way to get a 20 percent reduction in lung cancer mortality with a 30 percent adherence rate." He added, "Lung cancer screening targets a unique population that likely requires substantial engagement efforts to achieve outcomes." Shared decision making can foster patient autonomy and trusted relationships with clinicians that can improve adherence to screening, he said.

Mazzone added that many clinicians do not have experience with shared decision making. "We have to learn from others and I am sure, over time, we will evolve our shared decision-making visit to be better than it is now," he said. Elyse Park, associate professor of psychiatry at Harvard Medical School, said that the shared decision-making discussion should be an opportunity to talk about risk broadly, including information about smoking-related diseases that may be identified with lung cancer screening, as well as the risk of smoking on all health outcomes, not just on the risk for lung cancer.

Mazzone noted that most shared decision-making consultations are half an hour long and give patients a chance to ask questions or express concerns, "but although there are a few who ask a lot of questions, many think 'I am just going to do whatever my doctor said to do, no matter what you present to me' and they may not find it time well spent." Studts reported on a study that explored what influences patients' decisions to undergo lung cancer screening. Highest on the list of influences was a clinician's recommendation as well as cost. Access to screening was somewhat less of an influence, and the benefits and risks of screening, such as the false-positive rate and lung cancer mortality reduction, had the least influence on patients' decision making (Studts et al., 2012).

Amy Copeland, director of medical outreach at the Lung Cancer Alliance, added that there is a need for clarity on who can conduct the shared decision-making visit, when it can be conducted, how to bill for it, and how screening programs know that the visit has occurred. "There are still all these questions that our screening centers are struggling with on a day-to-day basis that we do not always have clear answers for," Copeland said. She has heard from screening centers about inconsistencies in codes that private payers are using for shared decision making and lung cancer screening, and there are also challenges with making sure all of the CMS requirements are met. "They want to do this well and just need a little more guidance to be able to do it well," she noted.

Chin said that CMS purposely defined the clinician who could provide counseling and shared decision making broadly to improve access, and can include a physician, physician's assistant, or certified nurse specialist. "It comes down to who is most responsible for these types of services for a particular individual, which usually is primary care, but a specialist like a pulmonologist or cardiologist may be the provider a particular beneficiary sees most often," he said.

Volk and Susan Schneider, associate professor at the Duke University School of Nursing and president of the Oncology Nursing Society, suggested that nurses could conduct the counseling and shared decision-making visit because they are trained to provide patient education and communication and often conduct informed-consent discussions for clinical trials. Volk added that decision coaches (usually nurses trained in conveying information and communicating with patients) could also be used to implement effective shared decision making. Studts added that his institution does not indicate a specific health care professional for the shared decision making: "We use the individual who has the passion, the drive, and the dedication to do it and to do it well, more so than focusing on any discipline," he said.

Chin added that a screening center may not be the best place to provide shared decision making, and perhaps there should be some separation between those who provide screening and those who order it. He noted that this is the first time CMS has required a shared decision-making visit prior to screening in order to provide coverage of the screening. Volk reiterated this, saying, "This is our first national experience with shared decision making being tied to a policy. We are in the midst of a national experiment right now."

Patient Decision Aids

Volk noted that shared decision making can be enhanced with clinician training, decision coaches, and reimbursement policies that foster shared decision making, practice redesign, and the use of patient decision aids. Hoffman added that patient decision aids can foster engagement in the process, especially since a study found that many primary care clinicians may not have experience with shared decision making (Volk and Foxhall, 2015). "They are a good way to make sure both the patients and providers understand what is going on," he said.

CMS recommends that clinicians provide patient decision aids when counseling patients about lung cancer screening. These aids are tools that help patients think about their choices by providing relevant information about options and their tradeoffs in a standardized way, according to Volk. "They support people to forecast what it might be like if they decide to go down one path versus another," he said, including the option of declining an intervention.

Volk added that patient decision aids are not designed to advise people to take one option over another, and they do not replace clinician consultations; rather, they are adjuncts to clinical encounters (Elwyn et al., 2010). "Shared decision making is a process. Patient decision aids are tools to help facilitate that process, but they do not ensure that shared decision making happens. It is not enough just to give a patient a decision aid and say 'read this' and then claim shared decision-making victory." Studts agreed: "I am very concerned that we are going to see patients being given aids with really no conversation or a very subpar conversation going on." Studts also emphasized that decision aids "are not designed to increase uptake [of lung cancer screening], but to help people make informed choices, which has some very important implications for long-term adherence."

Studts noted that decision aids can be used at various phases of the screening process to meet different needs. Some tools promote awareness or are preconsultation tools, which may help someone prepare for a discussion with their clinician. Other tools could be implemented to facilitate and maintain adherence to recommended screening regimens. Hoffman added that the VA has a separate decision aid for use after lung cancer screening results are provided.

Volk reported on the evidence base for patient decision aids, noting that a systematic Cochrane Review found that, compared to standard care, patient decision aids improved decision quality across a number of outcomes (see Table 3).

"Patients learned something, became more knowledgeable about their

TABLE 3 The Effect of Patient Decision Aids Compared to Usual Care

Improves Decision Quality		Modifies Decisions	
↑	14% knowledge	↓	20% elective surgery
↑	79% accurate risk perceptions	↓	14% prostate-specific antigen testing
↑	50% better match between values and choices	↑	18% colorectal cancer screening
↑	Patient–practitioner communication		
↑	41% help undecided to decide		No/minimal effect on anxiety, depression, regret, consult length, or health-related quality of life.
↓	6% decisional conflict		
↓	33% passive participation in decision making		

SOURCES: Volk presentation, June 20, 2016; Stacey et al., 2014.

own personal risk, and their preferences seemed to align with their decisions. They helped people who were undecided make decisions," Volk said. Decision aids had no or minimal effect on anxiety, depression, or regret, Volk added. Decision aids also influence the choices that people make, such as reducing uptake of elective surgeries and increasing effective cancer screening interventions (Stacey et al., 2014). "We do not know how patient decision aids are going to play out for lung cancer screening," Volk noted. "We have yet to see the evidence for them."

He said there are efforts to certify patient decision aids in the United States because hundreds of such aids have been developed, and it is unclear whether the evidence and information included in the aids are complete, reliable, and trustworthy, especially with the potential for conflicts of interest among those developing patient decision aids (Volk et al., 2013). He reported that the International Patient Decision Aids Standards Collaboration (IPDAS) was formed to enhance the quality and effectiveness of patient decision aids by establishing a framework for improving their content, development, implementation, and evaluation. This group created checklists for patient decision aids, tools for evaluation, and minimal standards (Volk et al., 2013). Important dimensions of quality for decision aids are shown in Table 4. The ACA called for a national certification effort for patient decision aids, Volk noted, and the National Quality Forum recently held a workshop to build consensus around national standards for patient decision aids and to identify approaches to measuring the quality of decision making and developing measures to assess the impact of decision making, Volk reported.

Only one state, Washington, has implemented policy measures related to patient decision aids. The Washington State Health Care Authority

TABLE 4 Quality Dimensions for Decision Aids Defined by the International Patient Decision Aids Standards Collaboration

- Systematic development process
- Disclosing conflicts of interest
- Information about options, harms, benefits
- Up-to-date evidence
- Balancing presentation of information and options
- Presenting probabilities
- Clarifying values and preferences
- Use of patient stories
- Health literacy
- Coaching and guidance
- Measuring effectiveness
- Delivering aids on the Internet

SOURCES: Volk presentation, June 20, 2016; Elwyn et al., 2006.

has developed certification criteria for patient decision aids following the IPDAS standards, and their use increases legal protection to physicians who use them during the informed consent process.

Volk discussed two patient decision aids for lung cancer screening that were developed with funding from the Agency for Healthcare Research and Quality (AHRQ). One decision aid is designed to be used before a clinical encounter and completed by a patient. It provides information about lung cancer screening and eligibility, potential harms and benefits of screening, and what is important when making a decision to be screened. It also includes questions to ask a health care professional about screening and insurance coverage. The second decision aid is designed to be used when the patient meets with the clinician and provides a brief synopsis of the potential harms and benefits of lung cancer screening, important considerations in making a decision, and insurance information. In the component of the decision aid devoted to values clarification, patients answer explicit questions about how they feel about the importance of different factors (i.e., whether they are concerned about possible false positives) (AHRQ, 2016).

These decision aids use visuals and language to describe the potential harms and benefits of lung cancer screening. They list the signs and symptoms of lung cancer and remind patients that the best way to prevent lung cancer mortality is by not smoking, Volk noted. When the potential harm of radiation from the screening is discussed, it is accompanied by a graphic showing how the dose of radiation received in a lung cancer screening compares with background radiation in the environment, and radiation exposures with other types of medical imaging. "We are really not very good at telling patients how much radiation is too much. But we can tell them how it compares to other sources of radiation," Volk said.

Studts reported on another decision aid, Lung Cancer Screening (LuCaS) Choices,[8] which is a Web-based patient decision aid developed to help individuals make informed decisions about lung cancer screening that are consistent with their values and preferences. The aid has three major sections: knowledge, empowerment, and values clarification. In the knowledge section, patients are informed of the potential benefits and risks of lung cancer screening with LDCT. It also includes personal risk assessment and screening eligibility calculators according to the USPSTF and NCCN guidelines.

The empowerment section encourages patients to talk with their clini-

[8] See https://clinicaltrials.gov/ct2/show/NCT02790866 (accessed September 29, 2016).

cians about lung cancer screening and shared decision making, and helps promote the development of deliberative skills. It also includes a question prompt list from which they can select questions they wish to raise with their clinicians. The final values component helps patients explore their personal values and how they relate to lung cancer screening. He added that this decision aid is comprehensive and time consuming, so it is not designed to be implemented in a consultation with a provider. "It really targets public awareness and information seekers—people actually trying to understand this choice," Studts said. He is currently testing the effectiveness of LuCaS Choices in a study of participants from Kentucky and Florida.

CHALLENGES TO IMPLEMENTATION OF LUNG CANCER SCREENING PROGRAMS

Steven Blumenfrucht, medical director of the New York market for Aetna, reported that there has been relatively low uptake of lung cancer screening thus far, at least in Aetna's current experience. Aetna reimburses LDCT lung cancer screening for patients who meet the USPSTF eligibility criteria; however, claims for screening did not significantly increase after release of the USPSTF recommendation, or the CMS national coverage decision (see Figure 3).

Hoffman noted similarly low uptake of LDCT screening in surveys of primary care physicians in New Mexico, South Carolina, North Carolina, and Texas (Ersek et al., 2016; Hoffman et al., 2015; Lewis et al., 2015; Volk and Foxhall, 2015). He added that some clinicians were still ordering baseline chest X-rays for patients who smoke. While 73 percent of respondents in South Carolina reported discussing LDCT lung cancer screening with their patients, only 41 percent of physicians had referred more than one patient during the past year. In North Carolina, more respondents ordered chest X-rays (21 percent) than LDCT lung imaging (12 percent). In Texas, 56 percent of respondents said they were planning to offer lung cancer screening, but less than half of them said they were able to refer patients to a high-quality screening program, could routinely identify eligible patients, or were able to engage patients in shared decision making. Only 10 percent of respondents said there was a well-functioning lung cancer screening program available to their practice.

Several workshop participants described factors that can contribute to the low uptake of lung cancer screening, including clinician knowledge and concerns about screening, challenges of implementing screening pro-

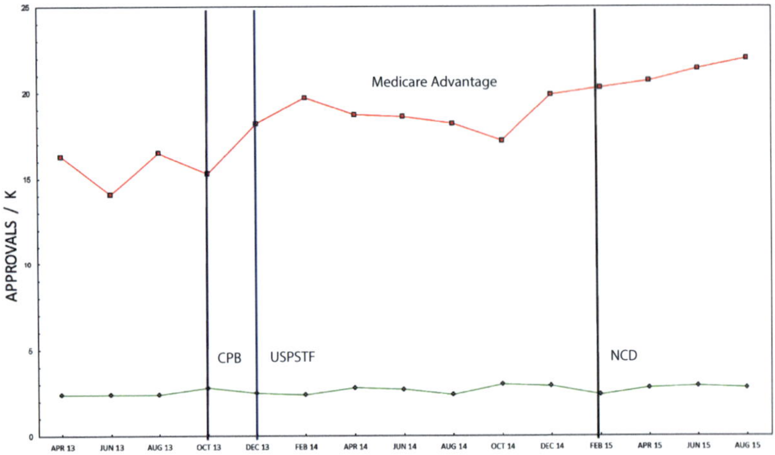

FIGURE 3 Aetna LDCT screening utilization. Aetna has not seen high uptake of LDCT lung cancer screening, either in the Medicare Advantage plans or in its commercial market.
NOTE: CPB = clinical policy bulletin; LDCT = low-dose computed tomography; NCD = National Coverage Determination; USPSTF = U.S. Preventive Services Task Force.
SOURCE: Blumenfrucht presentation, June 21, 2016.

grams in clinical practice, a lack of patient awareness or access to screening programs, and the unique challenges of reaching patients at high risk of lung cancer.

Clinician Awareness and Concerns About Lung Cancer Screening

Several participants noted that most individuals are referred to lung cancer screening by their primary care clinician. "Primary care is a critical component because these are the initial providers who talk with patients about the screening and assess their eligibility. They also usually provide referrals for the follow-up of positive findings and write orders for LDCTs that might be needed in the future," Kim said. However, clinicians may not be fully knowledgeable about lung cancer screening, or may have concerns about the intervention. Hoffman highlighted several areas of clinician concern regarding the implementation of lung cancer screening in clinical practice, including: skepticism about the evidence base and clinical practice guidelines, uncertainty regarding insurance coverage, and medical liability.

Hoffman interviewed family medicine clinicians in urban and rural areas of New Mexico, and found that they had limited awareness of NLST results 1 year after the USPSTF recommended lung cancer screening (Hoffman et al., 2015). A 2015 survey of primary care physicians in South Carolina found that only 41 percent of respondents believed LDCT screening reduced lung cancer mortality (Ersek et al., 2016). In a 2013 study of primary care physicians in North Carolina, only 42 percent rated screening as very or moderately effective in reducing lung cancer mortality, and many believed that lung cancer screening is less effective than screening for breast or colorectal cancer (Lewis et al., 2015). Surveyed clinicians were also concerned about the possible harms from screening, such as radiation exposure, risk from invasive diagnostic procedures and other interventions related to incidental findings, as well as the psychological stress of screening due to false positives, Hoffman reported. A common concern among primary care clinicians is that the false-positive rate of LDCT lung cancer screening is too high, he said.

Hoffman noted a lack of awareness of lung cancer screening guidelines among primary care clinicians. In surveys in North Carolina, South Carolina, and Texas conducted from 2013 and 2015, between 49 and 86 percent of survey respondents were aware of the lung cancer screening guidelines (Ersek et al., 2016; Lewis et al., 2015; Volk and Foxhall, 2015). In particular, there was low awareness of how frequently screening should be conducted and the age at which it should be stopped.

Some respondents in New Mexico noted that the USPSTF gave lung cancer screening a B recommendation, and it is largely based on a study of clinical trial participants who are not representative of New Mexico's population. Some respondents also pointed out that the clinical practice guidelines call for up to 25 years of annual screening, but the basis of this recommendation was less than 7 years of study follow-up in NLST. Respondents also expressed concern that the USPSTF recommendations may change, a concern that Hoffman agrees is valid; for example, new evidence could potentially lead to changes in the length of the screening interval following a negative screen, the use of risk-based modeling to identify high-risk individuals, or new management strategies to reduce the rate of false-positive results (Katki et al., 2016; Kovalchik et al., 2013; Patz et al., 2016). Clinicians also expressed concern in several surveys that lung cancer screening is not cost-effective, Hoffman reported, with some clinicians in New Mexico suggesting that the resources for lung cancer screening might be better allocated for smoking cessation interventions.

The American Academy of Family Physicians (AAFP) typically incorporates the USPSTF recommendations in its clinical practice guidelines, but decided that the evidence base for lung cancer screening is currently insufficient, noted Kelly Latimer, program director at the Naval Hospital Pensacola Family Medicine Residency. She added that this does not mean that the evidence will always be insufficient for recommending lung cancer screening. "The PROSPR [Population-based Research Optimizing Screening through Personalized Regimens] and NELSON trials will provide more data and then the AAFP will probably reevaluate lung cancer screening," she said (NIH, 2016; Yousaf-Khan et al., 2016). "It is just that it has not been proven in the real world. . . . We are not convinced yet."

Hoffman added that medical liability concerns could also influence implementation of lung cancer screening. Some clinicians may be worried about the legal implications of not offering lung cancer screening if they think a specific patient may not benefit, or if they have provided adequate shared decision making for informed consent. He suggested that clinicians use good documentation to describe the decisions and conversations about lung cancer screening.

Wood said that another challenge is the social stigma associated with smoking. "There is a little blame-the-victim mentality about lung cancer," LeFevre added, with society faulting individuals who smoke for developing lung cancer, even though the tobacco industry has promoted nicotine addiction: "We live in a society that does everything it can to get people addicted. Once we hook people on tobacco, it is hard to quit." Lathan agreed, noting the pervasive effect of tobacco companies, and added that many middle and high school students still recognize the Joe Camel cartoon, even though it has not been used in tobacco advertising since 2007. Kramer added, "Often a 15-year-old has made a choice [to smoke] not recognizing all the downstream effects, and 30 days later they no longer have a choice."

Lathan noted that medical students and residents often ask him how he can be inspired to treat lung cancer patients when their cancer was likely caused by smoking. He responds to students: "If somebody breaks their leg skiing, you do not say to them, 'Why did you go down a hill at 80-miles-an-hour on waxed plastic?' Instead you fix what you can."

Park noted that after her study results on the proportion of patients with colorectal and lung cancer who continued to smoke after their cancer diagnosis was publicized, of more than 400 comments posted online, only

1 comment referred to the patients with colorectal cancer who continued to smoke (Park et al., 2012). She emphasized that all of the commentary focused on lung cancer patients who smoked: "I think that is really revealing. We need to have conversations at the time of shared decision making, at the time of screening, and following screening about the different communication factors at the patient and physician levels and external factors like stigma."

Mills added that stigma can definitely pervade the care that patients with lung cancer receive, including her mother's care. "Thirty-five years ago, I was defending my mother's dignity as she was fighting for her life and here we are today still talking about the impact of stigma for people who smoke. We need to embrace them and say, 'You have made choices and now we have to help you.'"

Another participant pointed out that younger clinicians do not appreciate how prevalent smoking once was among older generations, and that there is a need for empathy and understanding of the environmental context. Smith added that clinicians need to recognize the influence of addiction: "The average physician who never smoked does not know what an addiction is like." They may tell patients, "You will quit when you are ready" or "You could quit it if you really wanted to," he said, "even though studies show how unhelpful it is to belittle people trying to quit smoking by making these remarks." Studts added: "When I work with providers on tobacco treatment implementation, I often ask them, 'What do you do in your daily life that you technically fail at 90 to 95 percent of the time and that you continue doing?'" He hopes this helps clinicians to understand the difficulty of quitting and to be better listeners when patients express their frustrations about trying to quit, and that clinicians can empathize with the challenge, but also reinforce the importance of continuing to make the effort. Park added that clinicians should not get frustrated when their patients who smoke fail to quit smoking after they refer them to cessation treatment, but instead recognize that not all patients will take action in this regard. If a patient is not ready to quit, she added that a clinician's role is to ask that they think about it.

Incorporation of Lung Cancer Screening in Clinical Practice

Some workshop participants also discussed issues that may hamper greater uptake of lung cancer screening in clinical practice, including

- A lack of time and competing demands;
- The need for tools, training, or personnel to conduct shared decision making;
- A lack of high-quality screening facilities available; and
- Difficulty in determining patient eligibility.

Hoffman noted that primary care clinicians often have many considerations during clinical visits, including management of chronic illnesses, acute problems, and preventive services. One study found that primary care physicians with a practice of 2,500 patients would have to spend more than 7 hours per day to implement all the preventive services recommended by the USPSTF (Yarnall et al., 2003). "There is a time cost," Hoffman said, and noted that a lack of time and competing demands may prevent clinicians from discussing lung cancer screening with their patients.

The complexity of lung cancer screening may be another challenge, several participants noted. "Lung cancer screening is so much more complicated than your average screening test, not to mention the shared decision-making visit. In 20 minutes, I do not have time to adequately do that, given that I have to also take care of their diabetes. . . . It is just not realistic. There are only 10 hours in a day and lung cancer screening tends to get lost in the whirlwind of everything else that needs to be done," said Latimer.

Clinicians and practices may not have the skills or the time to discuss lung cancer screening with patients, Hoffman noted. Clinicians surveyed agreed that such discussions and patient education were important, but said they also needed support for implementing shared decision making with patients, such as toolkits and decision aids, he reported. Clinicians in New Mexico were particularly concerned about informing patients with low literacy and limited proficiency in English. "These are complex issues. How do you explain to someone about abnormal results that do not clearly suggest cancer, but still warrant intensive surveillance? How do you explain to patients about the risks and downstream consequences of what is really involved in the screening program?" Hoffman asked.

Certain geographic areas may also lack high-quality screening facilities, Hoffman said. He pointed out that most guidelines specify for clinicians to refer their patients to a high-quality screening program, but the ACS recommends that if a patient is unwilling or unable to travel to a high-volume, high-quality screening and treatment center, then lung cancer screening is not recommended (Wender et al., 2013). Kazerooni noted that there are approximately 1,300 ACR-designated lung cancer screening centers, and that individuals can use the ACR accredited facility search to identify screening centers (ACR, 2016b).

A survey of family practice clinicians in Texas found that the clinicians were having trouble finding accredited screening programs, said Volk (Volk and Foxhall, 2015). These clinicians also wanted more information about the eligibility criteria for lung cancer screening, and were concerned about having tools available to engage patients in shared decision making.

Patient Access to Screening and Health Disparities

Several speakers pointed out that a major challenge to implementing lung cancer screening is the high proportion of individuals at high-risk for lung cancer who live in underserved communities, including individuals with lower educational achievement and socioeconomic status and racial and ethnic minorities. "You can list any health outcome and those who are poor, who speak a different language, and specifically African Americans seem to have poorer [health] outcomes," Lathan said, adding that African Americans are more likely than Hispanics or Caucasians to be diagnosed with and die from lung cancer (ACS, 2016).

Lathan and Smith said that disparities in access are contributing to some of the differences seen in cancer outcomes. Studies have shown that African Americans are less likely to obtain treatment for lung cancer at all stages, but when access to treatment is equivalent among African Americans and Caucasians, the disparities in survival disappear (Earle et al., 2002; Lathan et al., 2006). Smith added that disparities in access are still seen with screening for cervical, breast, and colorectal cancer, and he expected that "we clearly are going to encounter disparities in delivery of lung cancer screening."

Health disparities are also associated with differences in culture, Lathan noted (Albain et al., 2009; Echeverría et al., 2009; Kagawa-Singer et al., 2010; Williams and Mohammed, 2009). "We spend a lot of time on race, but we spend less time on socioeconomic status and very little time on culture, which really . . . has a dramatic impact" on health disparities and outcomes, Lathan said. He surveyed African Americans about their lung cancer beliefs, and found a reluctance to seek care due to fear, fatalism, and mistrust, as well as a lack of knowledge about the risks and outcomes of lung cancer. Patients wanted more help with smoking cessation and compassion from their clinicians (Lathan et al., 2015). One person interviewed suggested that the best way for clinicians to motivate heavy smokers to quit is to take images of their lungs for every year that they keep smoking. Lathan found this surprising given that the results of the NLST had not yet been published when this study was conducted.

Lathan said that low income predicts both an increased risk of using tobacco as well as an increased risk of dying from lung cancer. Income is also directly related to lung cancer stage at diagnosis (ACS, 2016; Albano et al., 2007). Lung cancer screening may also be hampered by financial costs and transportation issues encountered by patients with lower incomes, Mills noted.

Mazzone noted that patient compliance with annual screening at the Cleveland Clinic went from 35 percent to 64 percent after insurance coverage was in place and the screening program was centralized. Lathan added that another study found little difference in lung cancer survival between Medicaid and uninsured patients, and that both of these groups have worse survival rates compared to those who have private insurance (Walker et al., 2014).[9] "This is a major issue," Lathan stressed, because the ACA expanded access to Medicaid insurance with the intent of improving patient outcomes.

Brawley noted that the Medicaid expansion might improve access to lung cancer screening for some, but might also contribute to worsened state-by-state health disparities. There are more than 2.5 million poor, uninsured adults who fall into the coverage gap resulting from the 19 states that did not opt to expand their Medicaid programs (KFF, 2016). More than 90 percent of adults in this coverage gap reside in the southern United States, and Brawley noted that the states that have expanded Medicaid coverage tend to have fewer health disparities than states that did not (KFF, 2016). In addition to inadequate coverage for health care services, including cancer screenings, Brawley noted that cancer outcomes already vary greatly from state to state. For example, Brawley said that while the U.S. mortality rate from colorectal cancer has been declining over the past 25 years, 10 states have not seen reductions. In Mississippi, for example, there has been no decline in colorectal cancer mortality over the past 25 years. Twelve states have had less than a 10 percent decline in breast cancer mortality, while the national rate has declined more than 40 percent, Brawley reported.

Lathan added that even in Massachusetts, which has expanded Medicaid, African-American women still have greater breast cancer mortality.

---

[9] Cause-specific survival was defined as the time between diagnosis and death resulting from the primary cancer.

The state has restrictions on when and where Medicaid patients can receive screening that might be influencing outcomes, he said. "We put the most restrictions on our most vulnerable patients," he stressed.

There is also concern about whether patients have adequate insurance and/or finances to cover downstream diagnostic testing and treatment when lung cancer screening indicates that further evaluation is needed. Hoffman said screening patients for lung cancer is unethical if they cannot access subsequent diagnostic testing and treatment.

OVERCOMING IMPLEMENTATION CHALLENGES

Several workshop participants proposed suggestions for overcoming challenges to lung cancer screening implementation.

Clinician and Practice Strategies

Hoffman suggested clarifying the roles of primary care clinicians in lung cancer screening, including their responsibility for identifying appropriate patients, ensuring shared decision making, and overseeing appropriate follow-up. But identifying patients who are eligible for screening can be difficult. Some electronic medical records (EMRs) do not identify smoking status in pack-years, Hoffman noted. Latimer agreed that the EMR she uses does not adequately capture smoking history. "EMRs need to be written to ask those questions that identify eligible patients," she said. Lathan added, "Our experience has been that only about 10 percent of people eligible for screening get referred for it because they do not know their pack-year history. We really work with primary care doctors to try to address this because we need a reliable tobacco history." The CMS documentation requirements state that EMRs should include the appropriate templates for assessment of pack-year history.

Clinicians need guidance about patients who may be at high-risk for lung cancer but who do not fit the USPSTF recommendations, Hoffman said. "Radon is a big problem and I am not sure what I am supposed to do with that," he noted.[10] In addition, NCCN and ACS recommend that

---

[10] Estimates suggest that radon is responsible for approximately 15,000 to 22,000 lung cancer deaths per year in the United States; while the majority of radon-related lung cancer deaths occur in people who smoke, approximately 10 percent of radon-related lung cancer deaths occur in individuals who do not smoke. The combination of radon

clinicians offer lung cancer screening to eligible survivors of tobacco-related head and neck cancers, but clinicians need guidance in selecting these patients and what information to provide. For positive screens, primary care clinicians also need guidance from their colleagues in radiology and pulmonology to ensure appropriate surveillance and referrals for additional diagnostic evaluations, Hoffman added.

Hoffman also noted that primary care clinicians need assistance and tools to facilitate effective shared decision making (see Box 3). "Even though everyone agrees that shared decision making is a good thing, we have not been trained in that. We might want to have designated patient navigators who can be trained to deliver consistent, high-quality shared decision making," Hoffman said. Bach added, "These shared decision-making conversations are best done in the context of a trusted relationship with a provider who knows the patient fairly well, understands their values and their comorbidities." Bach also acknowledged how difficult it is to find the time to incorporate these discussions into a busy primary care practice. "I do not send somebody for a mammogram or a colonoscopy without having a discussion about pluses and minuses. I think it is doable, but we need to help providers a lot," Bach said.

Hoffman stressed that the decision to undergo screening is complex: "If we want to make sure this is a meaningful and shared decision-making effort, we probably need to have people who are trained and doing this repeatedly. This is a high-stakes screening decision and we need to make sure that shared decision making is truly happening and not just being checked off in the box." LeFevre added, "Creating tools is probably the most important thing we can do to make it easy and straightforward. But the primary care physicians do not feel comfortable with the data, so the easy thing is to refer and assume that [shared decision making] is going to happen someplace else." However, LeFevre was concerned about a lung cancer screening program conducting the shared decision-making process: "I am fairly skeptical that somebody [who] works for a cancer screening program is going to counsel somebody in a truly unbiased shared decision-making way."

Hoffman noted that one way to facilitate implementation of lung cancer screening is the use of performance measurement. Blumenfrucht suggested that lung cancer screening could be incorporated into the Healthcare

---

gas and cigarette smoke exposure creates a greater risk of lung cancer than exposure to either factor alone (NCI, 2011).

BOX 3
Resources and Tools to Facilitate Implementation of Lung Cancer Screening

A number of resources and tools to help clinicians and patients discuss lung cancer screening were highlighted in workshop discussions. For example, Robert Volk, professor at the MD Anderson Cancer Center, described the toolkit form the Agency for Healthcare Research and Quality (AHRQ), which includes a two-page summary guide and clinician checklist. The guide summarizes the evidence about lung cancer screening, eligibility requirements from the Centers for Medicare & Medicaid Services (CMS) and the U.S. Preventive Services Task Force (USPSTF), and information about insurance coverage. The guide also provides resources for smoking cessation, issues to discuss with patients, and a link to lung cancer screening facilities accredited by the American College of Radiology (ACR) (AHRQ, 2016). Volk said the one-page clinician checklist conforms to the CMS criteria so that it can be readily adapted for electronic health records. It includes the pack-year calculation formula, describes the follow-up process to a shared decision-making visit, and lists other tools and resources, including tips on how to provide shared decision making, talking points for the clinical encounter, and teach-back examples to ensure patient comprehension.

Joanna Stoms, cancer plan manager at the Pennsylvania Department of Health, described their lung cancer screening toolkit. This online resource was developed for clinicians, patients, and caregivers. The clinician resources include the CMS criteria for lung cancer screening, as well as decision-making tools, a list of ACR-accredited lung cancer screening facilities, and an overview of insurance coverage for screening (Pennsylvania Department of Health, 2016). The toolkit also provides a list of risk factors associated with lung cancer, as well as copay assistance information and drug assistance programs for patients and caregivers.

Effectiveness Data and Information Set (HEDIS) (NCQA, 2016) or used as a National Quality Forum measure because clinicians would be more motivated to discuss lung cancer screening and provide referrals. But Latimer noted that a new measure would add another decision prompt in the medical record, which she said is "the bane of primary care."

Others were also concerned about incorporating lung cancer screening as a performance measure because it could be an incentive for inappropriate screening. Bach said he is concerned that people who are ages 70 to 80, are frail, and have a high number of comorbidities and limited life expectancy "are going to get rushed off to get a scan because somebody has made it a quality checkmark." LeFevre added, "My biggest nightmare is that it becomes a quality measure because they are the antithesis to shared decision making. When it becomes a quality measure, I will not get graded on how many people I counsel about cancer screening, but on how many [people receive lung cancer screening]."

Hoffman said that in order for primary care clinicians to embrace lung cancer screening, "we need to have confidence that it can be safely, efficiently, and effectively implemented." That will require more population-based data from the "real world," he said, as well as building capacity so all patients have access to high-quality screening programs. "Most providers we spoke to a couple of years ago in New Mexico were taking a 'wait-and-see' [approach to lung cancer screening]. I do not think we can do that anymore, and primary care providers need to be proactive in figuring out how this could work best for themselves and their patients," Hoffman said.

Patient Outreach and Information Needs

Latimer suggested improving outreach to patients "so they can self-identify and come to us, because they are the ones who know how much they smoke." Mills agreed and suggested enhancing awareness through public service and public health messaging. She also suggested that information be tailored to individual needs and health literacy abilities, both in their design and messaging.

Several participants suggested that patient education efforts could try to counter the myths about smoking, lung cancer, and screening. "Some patients at the VA actually thought that screening itself would protect them against lung cancer. There is also the idea of the lucky smokers who, despite having a heavy smoking history, had negative scans so they do not have to quit smoking," Hoffman said. Lathan noted that one study found that Caucasian former smokers have a greater understanding of their lung cancer risk than African American former smokers. He suggested targeting educational outreach to specific vulnerable communities. "If you are going to get to the community, you need to target the community and talk to them. We cannot just set up a program and then expect people to come," he said. Studts noted that when designing patient decision aid tools for lung cancer screening, he and his colleagues targeted difficult-to-reach, high-risk populations for assessing usability.

Studts said that messages to patients need to convey "a balanced presentation of potential benefits and harms and avoid fear-based appeals that might engender distrust and stigmatize the group and perhaps push them in the wrong direction." He stressed that people who are eligible for lung cancer screening "are different than our typical screening populations [for other types of cancer], so we need to think about them differently from the very beginning, to understand who they are when designing our programs to meet their needs and to support them." For example, Studts said focus groups with individuals who were long-term smokers found that they expressed concern about stigma and distrust of the screening process, which could impact the successful implementation of screening programs (Carter-Harris et al., 2015). Studts added that reaching eligible individuals at high risk for lung cancer will require a trusted relationship with health care clinicians involved in screening, in order to ensure long-term patient engagement and adherence to lung cancer screening. Along with this trusted relationship, Studts added that lung cancer screening programs need to leverage this opportunity to provide individuals at high-risk of lung cancer with evidence-based tobacco treatment strategies. He also suggested that information about other factors that increase the risk of lung cancer, besides smoking, be incorporated into the educational materials given to patients. "If people are making the effort to go through a process of seeking lung cancer screening because they are concerned enough about their risk of lung cancer, why not incorporate messages with regard to radon and second-hand smoke exposures and other things that could potentially reduce their personal risk of developing lung cancer or reduce the risk for members of their family?" Studts said.

Park reported that her study found that current smokers are more likely to feel uncomfortable with health information presented in terms of numbers and statistics, compared to former smokers. Current smokers in the study were less likely to agree that statistics helped them make decisions about their health. This finding should be considered when delivering information on lung cancer and screening during shared decision making, Park said.

Doria-Rose asked how best to convey the risks of lung cancer screening conducted in community settings because the post-operative mortality seen in patients in the community is nearly five times the rate seen in participants in the NLST, and community programs may not have the same level of quality as in the trial. "This brings up issues of informed consent. What happens to the patient? What is their risk of post-op death? Does it matter if they go to center A versus center B, and should the patient know this? Should quality control parameters be built in? Is that part of the patient decision? Because it could make a lot of difference where they wind up getting treated," he said. Massetti noted that patients often do not want to travel for screening or treatment, and asked whether clinicians should refer patients to centers that have documented lower mortality following surgical resections, even if they are farther away. She added that the Society of Thoracic Surgery has a database in which surgeons' outcomes are reported and these outcomes are available for patients to see. "It is a very crucial point that patients get the best treatment, not just the best screening," she stressed.

Patient Access to Lung Cancer Screening

Several participants made suggestions to improve patient access to lung cancer screening, including greater collaboration among federal, state, and community organizations; enhancing outreach, education, and services for underserved populations; and leveraging mobile technologies and telemedicine. "We have to have some planning for how we are going to deliver evidence-based care to the vulnerable populations that would benefit the most and who suffer the most from the disease," Lathan stressed.

Lisa Richardson, director of CDC's Division of Cancer Prevention and Control, added that one of CDC's guiding principles is health equity, and the agency is trying to identify people who need access to screening services and ensure they receive them. She emphasized that there is a need for access to high-quality services for vulnerable populations and that improving access is dependent on the quality of available services.

Fabrice Smieliauskas, assistant professor at the University of Chicago, expressed concern that some community providers would not be able to provide high-quality lung cancer screening, and if such screening is restricted to only high-quality centers, access would be further decreased for those high-risk populations that need the screening the most. "There is going to be this tradeoff between high-quality, comprehensive programs and access . . . we may want to consider being flexible about whether every component of a gold-standard screening program is met, especially for hard-to-reach populations," he said.

Smith described a pilot program within federally qualified health centers, called Links of Care, which inventories unmet cancer screening needs in a community and then asks for equitable donation of those services among the clinicians and institutions in a given area that could meet those needs. Smith added that Links of Care is being used in the context of lung cancer screening. "It is rather labor-intensive, but so far it is showing real promise," Smith said.

Lathan added that Delaware's experience with colorectal cancer shows the impact of a concerted, collaborative effort to improve access to screening and treatment. Delaware was able to substantially reduce racial disparities in colorectal cancer (Grubbs et al., 2013). Lathan said this experience showed what could be accomplished when "government, policy makers, and clinicians all came together. It is a commitment issue. If you have the will—political and intellectual—it can be done." Smith agreed, noting that New York was able to reduce disparities in the screening rates among racial and ethnic groups by using coalitions to advance progress. Copeland also described a statewide consortium of hospitals and community partners in Kentucky that are assessing opportunities to improve access to cancer screening in rural areas. She added that Maine and North Carolina have been experimenting with mobile screening for hard-to-reach populations. "We are in a really exciting time and looking at a lot of opportunities to improve access to care, and we will learn a lot from these projects," she said.

Smieliauskas added that eventually new innovations in lung cancer screening could potentially be used in place of LDCT screening to screen hard-to-reach-populations, noting that a blood test for circulating tumor DNA is being evaluated for detection of lung cancer. However, Smith said that most serum tests tend to be expensive and have lower sensitivity and specificity parameters. He added that imaging would still be required to confirm suspected positive test results. "Ultimately, I think you are going to have to build basic capacity for screening one way or another into all of these underserved areas," Smith said.

Copeland noted that more work is needed to ensure access to diagnosis and treatment for positive imaging results. "We require our screening centers to have referral pathways to a multidisciplinary care team because it is great to do screening well, but if you have someone who is diagnosed, you need to get them into treatment because that is the part that really [could] save their lives. So we need to look at creative ways of not just ensuring access at the screening end, but also ensuring that access on the treatment end," she said.

SCREENING PROGRAM CAPACITY

Several participants expressed concern that broad implementation of lung cancer screening would strain the existing capacity to conduct such screening. Joshua Roth, assistant member and scholar at the Fred Hutchinson Cancer Research Center, highlighted the need for evaluation of demand versus the supply of lung cancer screening programs, imaging equipment, and medical professionals. "It is really important to make sure supply meets demand and that we allocate those resources around the country as needed," he said.

Smieliauskas reported on efforts to estimate demand and capacity for lung cancer screening nationwide. Demand is calculated using national health survey data that can be used to assess the population eligible for screening and where they are located, as well as to estimate what proportion of eligible people would seek screening. Smieliauskas said that several datasets capture "potential pieces of the capacity puzzle," such as the location of Lung Cancer Alliance–affiliated screening facilities or those that are accredited by ACR. Workforce estimates (radiologists and thoracic surgeons) as well as the location and quantity of CT scanners can also be assessed (Edwards et al., 2014; Smieliauskas et al., 2014).

Smieliaukas estimated the capacity constraints of radiologists and CT scanners due to the projected increases in LDCT scans for lung cancer screening by assuming that 75 percent of individuals who meet NLST eligibility criteria will undergo screening (see Figures 4 and 5) (Smieliauskas et al., 2014). "There are potential geographic access problems, largely in rural areas of America," Smieliauskas said. He found that 33 of 800 broad health service areas in the United States have no CT scanners, and 67 do not have multislice CT scanners. When assessing CT scanning capacity by county, Smieliauskas found 32 percent of counties have no CT scanner (approximately 8 percent of all eligible individuals live in these counties). Nearly half of all counties lack multislice CT scanners, including those that would serve 1.1 million individuals eligible for lung cancer screening (11 percent).

"If we really want to achieve universal equitable screening in all areas of the country, that would involve big investments to add CT scanners, radiologists, and thoracic surgeons in rural areas to achieve the capacity needed for the smoking burden that exists in those areas," Smieliauskas said. He suggested that such an investment should require (1) a high bar of evidence indicating that the expected benefits of lung cancer screening would exceed harms, and (2) a consideration of the cost-effectiveness of screening.

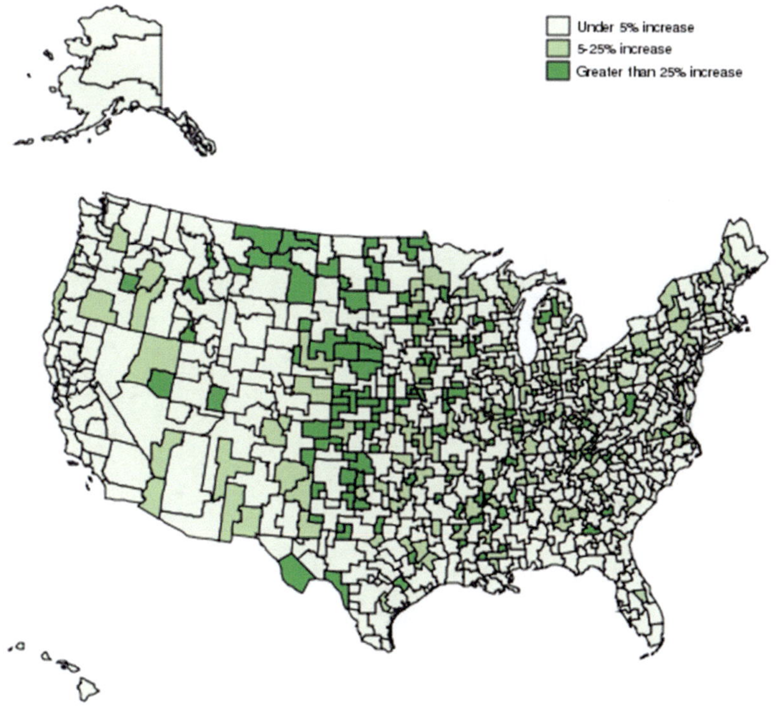

FIGURE 4 Percent change in LDCT scans performed by health service area. Although the majority of health service areas in the United States did not have high increases in the number of projected LDCT scans performed, the Midwest had the highest percentage increases.
NOTE: LDCT = low-dose computed tomography.
SOURCES: Smieliauskas presentation, June 20, 2016; Fabrice Smieliauskas, Heber MacMahon, Ravi Salgia, Ya-Chen Tina Shih, *Journal of Medical Screening* (21 and 4) pp. 207-215, Copyright © 2016 by SAGE Publications. Reprinted by Permission of SAGE Publications, Ltd.

Smieliauskas acknowledged that his assumption that 75 percent of eligible individuals would undergo screening could be an overestimate. In addition, he said estimated capacity needs are also are likely to be overestimates because they are based on the current population who smokes and current eligibility requirements for screening. The rate of smoking is expected to decrease in the future, and some estimates suggest that the

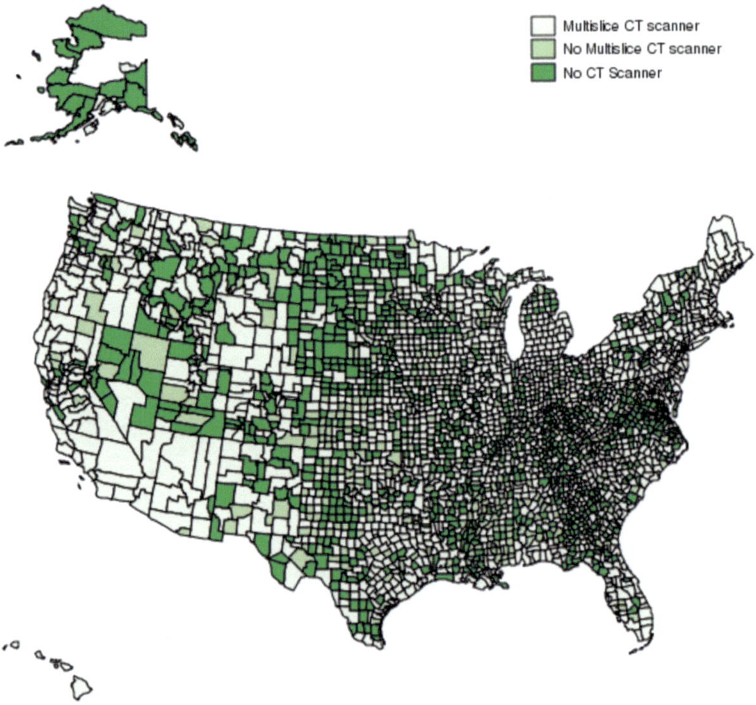

FIGURE 5 CT scanner capacity and geographic disparities in the United States by health service area.
NOTE: CT = computed tomography.
SOURCE: Smieliauskas presentation, June 20, 2016 (unpublished data).

number of people eligible for screening over the next 16 years could decrease by half (Edwards et al., 2014; Tramontano et al., 2016).

Smieliauskas noted that his estimates for capacity needs are based on instantaneous, rather than gradual, uptake of 75 percent of the eligible population. "Maybe we will have time to build up capacity to meet [the needs of] our target populations, but I expect it will go more quickly perhaps than that for previous cancers because screening is more mainstream now as part of cancer care," he said. Tammemägi noted that his own impression from the experience in Canada is a slow uptake of lung cancer screening. "There has been more gradual growth, which has been acceptable and easier to handle," he said.

To avoid overinvestment in capacity, Smieliauskas suggested applying some small-scale and cost-conscious strategies. For example, lung cancer screening could perhaps be conducted by community-based primary care clinicians and radiologists, with referral to comprehensive screening centers if there is a suspicious finding in the initial scan. Smieliauskas added that some pilot projects are assessing teleradiology, computer-aided detection, and volumetric nodule analysis to help address radiology workforce capacity limitations in some communities.

STRUCTURING LUNG CANCER SCREENING PROGRAMS

William Black, professor of radiology at the Dartmouth-Hitchcock Medical Center, outlined the steps involved in establishing a radiology program for lung cancer screening. Kim and Mazzone also described their experiences in establishing programs within the VA and at Cleveland Clinic, respectively, and the lessons learned from those experiences.

Program Set-Up

Black said the first step in establishing a lung cancer screening program is to assess institutional support. "This is critical—you must get complete buy-in from the radiology chairperson, primary care, lung cancer specialists, smoking cessation specialists, thoracic surgeons, pulmonologists, oncologists, and hospital and clinic administration," he said. Institutions should allot a fraction of a radiologist's time to organize the program and provide additional personnel, "because there is no radiologist who is going to be doing all the things that need to be done to make a lung cancer screening program viable," Black said.

He said that the individual developing the screening program needs to generate a plan that includes

- Creating an interdisciplinary team of primary care clinicians, pulmonologists, and other lung cancer specialists;
- Acquiring or creating shared decision-making materials;
- Creating a system for patient flow and follow-up that includes capturing patient data within the EMR;
- Creating a business plan; and
- Obtaining institutional funds to hire new personnel and allocating current employees' time to run the program.

A program coordinator is crucial "because you cannot implement lung cancer screening properly if you do not have somebody dedicated to this task," Black noted. A program coordinator (along with an administrative assistant) would oversee and perform several duties, including reviewing all requests for the screening and making sure they are appropriate, scheduling all screening procedures, managing a phone line dedicated to messages from patients and clinicians related to screening, and managing a database that tracks all information about lung cancer screening at the site and that can be submitted to a national registry. Black added that the radiology department should have an administrator who would oversee lung cancer screening operations and manage its budget.

Black said that assistance from a computer programmer would be needed to set up an image archiving and communication system, EMRs, and lung cancer screening databases. EMRs need to properly assess and document patient eligibility, shared decision making, and smoking cessation efforts and enable clinicians to order lung cancer screening tests. Scheduling the screening and any needed follow-up exams should also be integrated into EMRs, he said.

Radiologists interpreting lung cancer screening results should undergo training to meet the qualifications for doing such screening, Black said. Other radiology qualifications include developing a screening protocol, acquiring an ACR lung cancer screening designation, and enrolling in the ACR lung cancer screening registry to meet CMS requirements for reimbursement. A lung cancer screening reporting template, ideally based on the ACR Lung Imaging Reporting and Data System (Lung-RADS), needs to be developed for reading the lung images, Black said.

Software that can be used to build a lung cancer screening database would have to be purchased, which is "a pretty big barrier in terms of cost and time," Black said. This software can cost between $10,000 and $100,000 and requires extensive training. "It is a good idea that we have this database, but most radiology departments would not really have any experience setting up one, and it is very costly and unprecedented. We do not have these requirements for any other test in radiology," Black added. Final preparations involve making sure hospital and clinic billing systems are set up for lung cancer screening and ensuring that these departments are prepared to answer questions that clinicians or patients may have.

Daniel Sullivan, professor emeritus at the Duke University School of Medicine, pointed out that radiology departments have gained a lot of experience over the past 20 years developing breast cancer screening programs, which have many of the same elements and conceptual issues as lung cancer screening. He noted that, for many breast imaging centers, there is an efficient time frame from a positive screening result to when diagnosis and treatment occur, due to close collaboration among radiologists, primary care clinicians, breast cancer surgeons, and other clinicians. "There is no reason to think that this cannot be [achieved] in lung cancer screening. The radiology departments can develop these collaborations and operate very smoothly and effectively," he said.

Lessons Learned

Several presenters described their experiences with lung cancer screening programs and lessons that could be shared to improve implementation. "Development of an effective, high-quality lung cancer screening program requires recognition that this is not just a test, but a multi-faceted program," Mazzone stressed, noting the need for multi-disciplinary teams with broad expertise, shared vision, and administrative support. Kim pointed out that the commitment to lung cancer screening among primary care clinicians was quite variable in the VA pilot program. "It took a lot of finessing on the local level to see where each provider was and to work with them. A strong partnership was really essential from informatics through primary care," she said.

Kim also noted the significant resources needed to implement a systematic approach to lung cancer screening, including radiology equipment and staff; a multidisciplinary team from radiology, oncology, surgery, and pulmonology; and information technology support for the development of a tracking system. In addition, a lung cancer screening program requires primary care clinical staff time for initial training, the conduct of shared decision making, and follow-up of findings. Aberle added, "You have to use dedicated staff and tracking software that is expensive, but commercially available for these screening programs."

Black also highlighted the need for dedicated personnel, software support, and time to ensure that eligibility criteria are met; shared decision making occurs; screening results are communicated; and program outcomes are tracked. He said that it can be time consuming to ensure that individuals meet eligibility criteria and to sufficiently document shared decision making in EMRs.

Doria-Rose stressed "the need for a large amount of coordination within lung cancer screening programs, as well as the need for IT [information technology] tools that can improve the process of acquiring high-quality data from screening." Kim noted that a survey of clinicians who participated in a VA pilot program said that a lung cancer screening coordinator was an essential position for determining patient eligibility, tracking and ensuring appropriate follow-up management and care, and communicating among the patient and all clinicians involved in screening process (see Box 4).

Several participants suggested centralizing aspects of lung cancer screening. Black said that centralizing the eligibility assessment and the shared decision-making process could reduce the workload for primary care clinicians and radiologists. "The advantage of having some type of national program for determining eligibility and for decision making would be that it would be done in a much more consistent fashion. Personally, I think it is terribly inefficient to try to train every single provider how to do shared decision making." He added that eligibility assessments and shared decision making are expensive in terms of time and "our primary care doctors are overloaded with other things to do."

Smith also noted that the identification and recruitment of eligible individuals is enormously stressful on primary care clinicians and places a lot of demands on them. "We are challenged to perhaps ask if there is an alternative way to engage primary care, but relieve them from many of the responsibilities of recruiting adults for lung cancer screening and following them. How do we keep them in the loop, but perhaps systematize this in

BOX 4
Department of Veterans Affairs Lung Cancer Screening Pilot

Many veterans are at increased risk for lung cancer because the prevalence of smoking in this population is high, said Jane Kim, acting chief consultant for preventive medicine at the National Center for Health Promotion and Disease Prevention of the Department of Veterans Affairs (VA). To provide guidance on the implementation of lung cancer screening in the veteran population, the VA conducted a 3-year lung cancer screening demonstration project, completed in 2015. Eight VA sites participated in the project, which focused on implementation issues, and not on patient outcomes, Kim stressed.

BOX 4 Continued

Funding was provided to participating facilities for a clinical site coordinator. The program funded the development of electronic tools to support screening, and the pilot used smoking cessation programs already widely used in the VA. Participating sites were chosen based on expertise in lung nodule detection and lung cancer treatment, but did not include locations where lung cancer screening research was conducted.

To determine patient eligibility, the VA built electronic decision-support tools tailored to the VA's medical record system. These tools helped primary care clinicians to determine smoking history, age, and other requirements, and had built-in prompts to select patients for lung cancer screening. As part of the pilot, the VA also developed patient education materials to aid shared decision-making conversations, both at the time of initial counseling, as well as after the screening result was determined. The VA developed an electronic method to track patients in the screening program and enter their data into a database that was integrated into the VA's electronic medical records. The coordinators used this database and electronic templates to document care in the medical record and to ensure patients were not lost to follow-up. The VA also developed a radiology dictation guide based on the modified Fleischner Criteria because the American College of Radiology (ACR) Lung Imaging Reporting and Data System (Lung-RADS) was not yet available.

After 3 years, the VA evaluated their demonstration project and found that smoking history could be determined in 61 percent of primary care patients who met age and life expectancy criteria for lung cancer screening. Of those patients, 32 percent met smoking history criteria. Approximately three-quarters of these patients were deemed not appropriate for the screening by their clinician, based on their comorbidities and other factors. Fifty percent of the eligible patients did not agree to or did not complete lung cancer screening. Sixty percent of veterans screened had positive tests requiring tracking or further workup, and 40 percent had incidental findings. Kim estimated that only about 10 percent of the incidental findings were significant enough to require clinical follow-up.

Based on their evaluation of the demonstration project, the VA estimates that about 750,000 of its patients could be offered lung cancer screening, which would require significant resources to provide. The VA is currently considering the results of the pilot and how to move forward with lung cancer screening, Kim said. "My leadership has received these findings and is currently considering what to do in light of the significant resource needs," Kim said.

another way?" he asked. Smith suggested state-level engagement may be needed to address all of the challenges in lung cancer screening that may not easily be addressed at the national level.

Kim added that the VA pilot found a need for a central database and/or registry that communicated with the VA's EMRs. A designated national lung cancer management team could provide ongoing guidance, support, and oversight, including communication and system-wide implementation of practice updates such as Lung-RADS, as well as changes in screening guidance and coding. "People look to a national VA office to tell them what to do or to help them. Without that national guidance, each facility feels a little bit lost at times," she said. Providing that national support would require investing at the national VA level in a staff dedicated to aiding implementation of lung cancer screening. "Even if we did this on a smaller scale, you would still need to have some centralized support to make sure that things are being done according to a national standard," Kim said.

Mazzone noted that Cleveland Clinic's lung cancer screening program became more centralized in order to improve efficiency and effectiveness (see Box 5). Clinicians can now only order a consult to the screening program. Determining eligibility, shared decision making, ordering the scan, follow-up of screening results, and smoking cessation counseling occurs at the program level rather than at the clinician level. "It is not that the provider cannot still talk about the risks and benefits of screening or provide their own smoking cessation counseling, but now we take responsibility for doing that ourselves," he said.

Mazzone added that Cleveland Clinic started small and relatively slowly in order to learn "how to put together the program and to address its quality issues. Clearly now it is time for us to be providing the service more broadly." He added that the shared decision-making visit occurs at Cleveland Clinic's main campus, but he frequently receives calls from clinicians who say that their patients are not willing to travel to the main campus. "Growing beyond Cleveland Clinic's walls is something we would be open to, and sharing our experience, but we have to get it right in our region next. We are a little nervous about whether regionalizing will [endanger] our main campus program. Do we have to [set up] all that infrastructure out in the region, and are we still going to have the same volumes on the main campus? We will learn and adjust as needed," Mazzone said.

Black noted that a large workload component of lung cancer screening is directly related to the radiologist's task of searching for nodules and reporting findings. To make screening more time efficient, Black suggested

BOX 5
Cleveland Clinic's Lung Cancer Screening Program

Peter Mazzone, director of the Lung Cancer Screening Program at Cleveland Clinic, said that this program follows the Medicare or U.S. Preventive Services Task Force (USPSTF) guidelines for eligibility. The program is attempting to develop a research arm for individuals who are at high risk for lung cancer but do not meet current eligibility criteria. Symptomatic patients are instead referred for diagnostic evaluation. For patients with serious comorbidities, Mazzone said that discussions are held with pulmonologists and cardiologists to help determine the appropriateness of lung cancer screening.

To reach the eligible individuals, the Clinic developed a multifaceted approach aimed at clinicians and patients. Information about the screening is provided in grand rounds presentations, health system newsletters, on-hold messages, Web-based resources, decision aids, health fairs, letters to patients, pamphlets, a call line, and journal articles. "There is never enough education of the people who are using the program," Mazzone stressed. The program also attempted to develop a reminder system for the clinic's electronic health record, and has mined patient data on this electronic database.

Although initially clinicians could order lung cancer screening, now they can only order a consult with the screening program. If a patient is eligible, the program schedules a shared decision-making visit for the patient, followed by a computed tomography scan, if they choose screening. Patients who are not eligible are notified about why they were considered ineligible. In the past year, the program had more than 1,100 consult orders placed, and only 56 did not meet qualifications (see Table at the end of Box 5).

Shared decision-making visits are conducted with a nurse practitioner who is trained as a counselor. After determining eligibility, the nurse practitioner shows patients a brief narrated slide show about the potential harms and benefits of the screening. The program also uses a shared decision-making tool developed by the University of Michigan to illustrate individual risks and benefits of the screening. In addition, the nurse practitioner prepares patients for results by discussing the likely findings and how they will be communicated to patients. Annual screening is also stressed, and patients who smoke are connected to local smoking cessation resources. A template note with extractable elements is used for documenting and reporting the shared decision-making visit. An

continued

BOX 5 Continued

analysis found that this visit improved patients' knowledge of the potential benefits and risks of lung cancer screening, and that some of that knowledge was long-lasting.

Cleveland Clinic follows the American College of Radiology (ACR) guidelines on lung cancer screening, and its radiologists track radiation doses to ensure they are below the recommended limit. Radiology results were initially provided within a structured report developed by Cleveland Clinic, but now the Clinic uses reporting formats from the ACR Lung Imaging Reporting and Data System (Lung-RADS), from which data can be automatically abstracted. A text-dictated section is provided for findings other than nodules. Patients with negative findings are informed of their results and reminded to return for their next annual screen, while those with serious findings are informed of their risk based on Lung-RADS criteria, as well as the process and timing for follow-up. All screening results are owned and followed-up by the program rather than the clinician, Mazzone noted, including scheduled consults and follow-up tests. Smoking cessation resources are also provided by the program.

Follow-up of abnormal nodule findings is completed in a centralized manner by the program and based on the care paths specified by Lung-RADS, with the program consulting guidelines and collaboration with relevant specialists to manage incidental findings. Biopsy and treatment decisions are discussed at a tumor board before they occur, Mazzone said. A management tracking system tracks patients' follow-up care.

Cleveland Clinic encourages patients' compliance with annual screens with monitoring through an internal registry, and by sending letters and making phone calls to patients, who are offered a shared decision-making visit at each screen. "We think a patient's knowledge will wane a little bit over time, and there may be new information we can present at this visit. We may also need to reassess their eligibility," Mazzone said. Another reason to repeat the shared decision-making visit is to provide another face-to-face opportunity to develop a relationship with the patient and to stress smoking cessation, he added.

To comply with the data requirements of the Centers for Medicare & Medicaid Screening (CMS), the program has an internal registry that automatically pulls data from the order set, the structured radiology report, the shared decision-making visit note, and the electronic medical record.

The lung cancer screening program was started at Cleveland Clinic's main campus, and all scans are provided at the main campus.

Recognizing that some patients do not want to travel to the main campus, the Clinic is starting to develop screening programs in five of its satellite health centers.

TABLE Cleveland Clinic Screening Program

	Before Program Centralization	After Program Centralization	Total
Number	667	441	1,108
Male to female ratio	2.0	1.6	1.9
Age (mean)	63.9	64.2	64.0
Outside age range	4.0%	0%	2.4%
Smoking history	C – 41%; 36.7 pack-years	C – 51%; 51.3 pack-years	C – 45%; 44 pack-years
Outside smoking history criteria	18.1%	0.2%	10.9%
Nodules	79%	90%; 70% ACR category 2, 11% ACR 3, 5% ACR 4	83%
Avoidable procedures	1	1	2
Smoking intervention	82%	100%	89%
Patients eligible for annual screening	85 of 240 (35%)	42 of 66 (64%)	127 of 306 (42%)
Lung cancers	9 (2 stage I)	2 (2 stage I)	11 (4 stage I)
Other cancers	6	1	7

NOTE: ACR = American College of Radiology; C = current smokers.
SOURCE: Mazzone presentation, June 21, 2016.

using computer-aided detection for finding lung nodules. "Some of the radiologist's search time could be greatly reduced by programs that can find small nodules so that radiologists could spend more of the time on the suspicious nodules rather than looking at normal lungs," Black said. He added that computer-aided diagnosis could also help with further characterization of nodules.

But Aberle noted that "whether we will be using semantic features, computational features, or some combination is still open for discussion because in the United States we are fairly early in implementing computer-aided diagnosis systems." Features that are described, as opposed to detected via a computer algorithm, are relatively insensitive to imaging techniques, but there is not great reader agreement on them, according to Aberle. "We need to develop an imaging atlas that will help calibrate readers across centers," she suggested, noting that image interpretation could use standardized terminology based on illustrated lexicons. She also suggested standard acquisition of images "because I believe that it will become part of the fabric of our screening programs." She noted that efforts are under way to reduce variants and determine which features of quantitative imaging can be reproducible across heterogeneous data.

Black also suggested that there could be improvements in automated structured reporting so that when a radiologist measures a nodule, that measurement would be automatically incorporated into a report, which could improve accuracy and efficiency. Kim pointed out that the VA lung cancer screening pilot identified a need for a standardized protocol for nodule tracking that could be shared by all VA institutions, as opposed to the site-specific tracking systems that were developed.

Smith suggested decision aids used in shared decision making should be standardized and routinely updated, so that they reflect the current knowledge about how best to express benefit, harm, and risk. Smith also stressed that "screening is a cascade of events, and if any one step in the process goes badly, you undo all the good you have done in the previous steps and you have not set the stage for the next ones. We have learned that screening works best when it is organized." He added, "Organized screening would have a system in place with rules, roles, and relationships defined so that every person can depend on what the other is supposed to do, evaluation is in place, and corrective action can be instituted when needed."

Aberle said that in comparison to the diffusion of breast and colorectal cancer screening, the diffusion of lung cancer screening programs has been rapid. "NLST had an explosive effect—it brought lung cancer screening to the foreground and we have had to hurry in order to be able to provide that service. I do not think we are there yet, or at least very few sectors are. But we would have the capacity to do it because the systems, the communication infrastructures, the nodule and tracking systems, and our ability to understand that we cannot handle this without an administrative and health care infrastructure that supports this are lessons we are learning really rapidly," she said.

Kazerooni added that "we have a long way to go in terms of awareness and education about lung cancer screening among the public and the health care community. It is going to take a village—many people at many levels to get to where we are now with breast cancer screening and to do it safely and effectively, but I have no doubt that we will get there. We should work toward high-quality screening so that people are having dinner conversations about lung cancer screening the way they have about breast cancer screening today."

ENSURING THE QUALITY OF LUNG CANCER SCREENING

Several workshop participants said that it is critical to ensure implementation of high-quality lung cancer screening programs in order to achieve the benefits seen in NLST. Smith said that CMS reinforces the focus on quality by reimbursing screening only if strict requirements are met. Doria-Rose emphasized that lung cancer screening is not a single test, but a complex process dependent on multiple steps, including eligibility assessment, shared decision making, performing the screening test, interpreting results, providing diagnostic follow-up exams when needed, and treating patients diagnosed with cancer. "Successful completion of each one of these steps is necessary for the maximal screening benefit to be realized," he said. "Conversely, breakdowns at any point in the process, including failure to screen, failure to detect abnormalities at screening, failure to follow-up the abnormalities appropriately, or failure to treat appropriately, are all going to lead to suboptimal outcomes. These failures can be due to patient noncompliance or they can be failures on the part of medical providers or health systems to recommend and conduct appropriate testing and treatment," he added.

Mazzone said that two pulmonary societies have defined essential components of a high-quality lung cancer screening program, including

- Who is offered lung cancer screening;
- How often and for how long to screen;
- How the computed tomography is performed;
- Lung nodule identification;
- Structured reporting;
- Lung nodule management algorithms;
- Smoking cessation;
- Patient and provider education; and
- Data collection (Mazzone et al., 2015).

Several workshop participants highlighted opportunities to improve the quality of lung cancer screening by focusing on eligibility, adherence to annual screening, smoking cessation services, image interpretation and management of findings, and monitoring screening program results over time.

Confirming Eligibility for Lung Cancer Screening

Several speakers noted that lung cancer scans are sometimes scheduled for people who do not meet current eligibility requirements, and they discussed opportunities to avoid this. Black noted that his program's coordinator would only schedule a screening after speaking with a patient and confirming that he or she meets eligibility requirements. The coordinator also ensures with this initial telephone call that the patient understands what is involved with lung cancer screening, including its potential benefits and harms. Aberle stressed, "Determining eligibility is a major problem and having referrals for patients who are ineligible according to current criteria is not a trivial problem. In those patients who do not satisfy the criteria, we do not really know the risk–benefit ratios and the screens are not a covered benefit. It is problematic and will require some degree of education." She applauded Cleveland Clinic's reliance on its own trained personnel to determine eligibility.

Maintenance of Annual Lung Cancer Screening

Copeland stressed the importance of adherence to annual lung cancer screening in order for it to be effective. "The adherence issue is huge. It is not enough to get a person in for that first scan because that is not going to be the scan that necessarily saves the person's life. It is getting that individual in over and over again that is key, and we are really wrestling with that and need to figure out ways to do it," she said. She reported that only 24 out of 400 Lung Cancer Alliance's lung cancer screening sites report 80 to 100 percent adherence rates for annual scans, and she suggested evaluating best practices for improving adherence.

Ensuring Access to Smoking Cessation Services

Jamie Ostroff, chief of the behavioral sciences service and director of the Tobacco Treatment Program at the Memorial Sloan Kettering Cancer Center, suggested developing a standard set of process and outcome measures related to smoking cessation services within lung cancer screening programs (see also section on smoking cessation and lung cancer screening). She added that these measures could be included when registering lung cancer screening sites "so we can ensure [that] we are providing high-quality tobacco cessation treatment in high-quality screening centers. There are policy and guidelines opportunities here."

High-Quality Image Interpretation and Management of Findings

Kazerooni reported on the ACR practice parameters for the performance and interpretation of lung cancer screening, which include fundamental practice parameters for performing screening CTs; the use of the Lung-RADS structured reporting and management tool; and referring patients to an ACR-designated lung cancer screening center under the CT accreditation program. ACR also developed a lung cancer screening registry in 2015, and CMS coverage requires participation in the registry. "Since the ACR is currently the only CMS-approved registry for facility reimbursement, and the ACR registry requires the use of Lung-RADS, if you are conducting lung cancer screening in the United States and want to be reimbursed [by CMS] as a facility or provider, you have to use Lung-RADS," Kazerooni said.

Lung-RADS is similar to the Breast Imaging Reporting and Data System (BI-RADS), which is used to structure reporting and management of breast cancer screening results and findings (ACR, 2016a). Lung-RADS defines categories of positive results and for each category provides a management recommendation. Lung-RADS measures the diameter of nodules rather than volume, which is measured with computer-aided diagnosis.

However, that technology is not yet widely validated or disseminated in the United States, according to Kazerooni, but is used more widely in Europe.

Lung-RADS attempts to lower the false-positive and overdiagnosis rates linked to lung cancer screening by raising the threshold size of suspicious nodules and categorizing other features of the nodules. Wood said a study demonstrated that if Lung-RADS is applied retrospectively to the NLST images, it diminishes the false-positive rate in the baseline scans by 52 percent and in the follow-up scans by 76 percent (Pinsky et al., 2015). However, Kazerooni added that this reduced false-positive rate is linked to a decrease in sensitivity by 8 and 15 percent for baseline and follow-up scans, respectively. Kazerooni noted that by increasing the size threshold, there is a tradeoff of potentially delaying diagnosis of a cancerous nodule: analysis of NLST results indicated that increasing the threshold diameter from 5 to 8 millimeters would increase missed or delayed cancer diagnoses from 1.0 to 15.8 percent, but it would also reduce the false-positive rate from 65.8 to 10.5 percent and substantially reduce the use of medical resources (Gierada et al., 2014). "What is the tradeoff here, how does it affect outcomes?" Kazerooni asked, adding, "We need to know more about this in the future."

Lung-RADS also took into account the revised adenocarcinoma classification scheme, which was a multidisciplinary and international effort that defined subtypes of adenocarcinoma and correlated imaging with pathologic findings. "We know that not all of these cancers will impact the human in whom they live," she said, and noted that the new classification scheme designates some lesions as pre-cancerous lesions.

Based on the size and features of nodules, Lung-RADS has a structured reporting and management scheme (see Table 5). Nodule size is characterized by whether the nodule is new or is growing. Nodule consistency considerations are whether the nodule is solid, part solid, or non-solid (a non-solid nodule is also referred to as ground glass nodule), as well as whether the nodule includes certain benign features, such as fat or calcifications. Some nodules may contain features that will need to be followed closely, each year or sooner, with CT or positron emission tomography (PET) imaging to see if they develop any signs of invasive cancer. In addition to imaging, some suspicious nodules may also require tissue biopsies.

Black noted how time consuming it is to examine a lung scan for nodules, let alone scrutinize those nodules detected for features indicative of invasive cancer. Each CT scan consists of more than 400 slices of 1-millimeter cuts, he said, adding "It can be really tricky to find the nodules when they are central, about the same size as blood vessels, and only apparent on one or two slices. It is not a trivial task." Based on one study, he estimates it takes about 20 minutes just to examine each scan to detect nodules, and additional time to categorize and report those nodules using Lung-RADS. As previously noted, Black suggested that a radiologist's search time could be greatly reduced by using computer-aided detection and diagnosis to detect and characterize nodules.

Aberle said that there are a number of commercially available software programs for computer-aided detection and diagnosis of solid lung nodules, and that some are approved by the Food and Drug Administration (FDA) for clinical use. She added that although use of such programs is the norm in European countries, adoption has been slow in the United States, mainly because of workflow issues, she suspects. In Europe, these analyses are run by radiologic technologists trained to use the program, so the workflow is more efficient. That may eventually be the model in the United States, she said. Computer-aided detection and diagnosis "is inevitable because once we begin to ramp up, even to 20 to 30 percent of the eligible population for screening, we are going to need to have those kinds of efficiencies in the workplace," she said. Some U.S. institutions are already using these technologies for lung cancer screening and reporting volumes as well as diameters, Aberle added.

Both Kazerooni and Aberle added that Lung-RADS may evolve to rely on three-dimensional measurements and computer-aided detection and diagnosis. "Volumetrics makes more sense as a way to measure nodule growth and I would certainly hope that Lung-RADS evolves from diameters to volumes over time," Aberle said. Kazerooni added, "Lung-RADS is not static, but dynamic and will iterate." But she stressed that "We have a lot to learn about the implications and use of computer-aided diagnostic tools and practice. Learning from the breast imaging world and then applying that to lung cancer screening will help us a lot."

Monitoring Results

To promote quality improvement in lung cancer screening programs, Lung-RADS facilitates data collection for the ACR registry, Kazerooni said. She reported that the ACR lung screening registry is the first and only nationwide lung cancer screening registry approved by CMS, and developed specifically in response to the CMS registry reporting requirement.

In addition to the CMS requirements, ACR requires outcomes in the registry to be reported 12 months after a screening, including diagnostic

TABLE 5 American College of Radiology Lung-RADS Structured Reporting and Management

Category	Description	Estimated Prevalence	Probability of Malignancy	Management
Incomplete 0	—	1%	n/a	Additional lung cancer screening CT images and/or comparison with prior chest CT examinations needed
Negative 1	No nodules and definitely benign nodules	90%	<1%	Continue annual screening with LDCT in 12 months
Benign Appearance or Behavior 2	Nodules with a very low likelihood of becoming a clinically active cancer due to size or lack of growth			
Probably Benign 3	Probably benign finding(s); short-term follow-up; includes nodules with low likelihood of becoming clinically active cancer	5%	1-2%	6-month LDCT

Suspicious 4A	Findings for which additional diagnostic testing and/or tissue sampling is recommended	2%	5-15%	3-month LDCT; PET/CT may be used when there is a ≥8 mm solid component
4B		2%	>15%	Chest CT with or without contrast, PET/CT and/or tissue sampling depending on the probability of malignancy and comorbidities. PET/CT may be used when there is a ≥8 mm solid component.

NOTE: CT = computed tomography; LDCT = low-dose computed tomography; Lung-RADS = American College of Radiology Lung Imaging Reporting and Data System; PET = positron emission tomography.
SOURCES: Kazerooni presentation, June 20, 2016, from ACR, 2014.

follow-up testing, tissue sampling and diagnosis, lung cancer diagnosis, and stage. The registry requires sites to enter data on all screened individuals, not just those covered by CMS, "to give us a true picture of screening and practice," she said. The registry enables tracking of patients over time, even if they move to a different clinician. "Our goal is to be able to follow those patients so we do not just get 1-year screening outcomes, but 2-, 3-, and 5-year screening outcomes effectively," Kazerooni said. For board certified radiologists, active participation in the registry meets the maintenance of certification requirement for practice quality improvement. Uptake of the registry has been very fast, Kazerooni reported.

Doria-Rose also described current NCI efforts to monitor lung cancer screening outcomes within community settings, including the lung cancer screening pilot within the Cancer Research Network (which includes the Henry Ford Health System, Kaiser Permanente Colorado, Kaiser Permanente Northern California, and Kaiser Permanente Southern California) and the PROSPR program. In 2014, the Cancer Research Network funded pilot efforts to develop infrastructure to monitor the risks and benefits of lung cancer screening within health systems, and to disseminate strategies to facilitate improved data collection. Doria-Rose added that there are plans to add lung cancer screening to the PROSPR program, whose objective is to promote coordinated, multidisciplinary, multilevel research to evaluate and improve screening processes in clinical practice (NIH, 2016).

SMOKING CESSATION AND LUNG CANCER SCREENING

Several workshop speakers discussed concerns and challenges in integrating smoking cessation services within lung cancer screening programs. The results of current integrated programs, and how best to incorporate smoking cessation counseling and resources into a lung cancer screening program, were both areas of active discussion.

Approximately half of all patients who undergo lung cancer screening are current smokers (Humphrey et al., 2013; Slatore et al., 2014), said Kathryn Taylor, professor of population sciences at Georgetown Lombardi Comprehensive Cancer Center. Experts agree that smoking prevention is the best way to prevent lung cancer, and lung cancer screening should not be a substitute for cessation. For example, the patient and physician guide explaining the NLST trial results stated that the most important thing that individuals can do is not to smoke:

> Regardless of your screening decision, avoiding cigarettes is the most powerful way to lower your chance of dying overall or suffering or dying from a variety of diseases, such as lung cancer, emphysema, heart or vascular disease. For example, at age sixty-five, 89 in 1,000 male current smokers will die of lung cancer in the next 10 years versus 4 in 1,000 never smokers. For women, the corresponding figures are 55 in 1,000 versus 5 in 1,000. For help quitting, call 1-800-QUIT-NOW. (NCI, 2016b)

"The difference in risk of lung cancer between getting screened and never smoking or stopping smoking is stark and not even the same order of magnitude," Kramer stressed.

However, there is an added benefit to quitting smoking even after screening has begun, said Christopher Slatore, associate professor of pulmonary and critical care medicine at Oregon Health & Science University. He reported on a study that found people undergoing lung cancer screening who quit smoking further decreased their risk of dying from lung cancer compared with those who did not quit (Pastorino et al., 2016). A modeling study also demonstrated the added mortality benefit of quitting smoking in addition to undergoing lung cancer screening (McMahon et al., 2012). Taylor and Studts said modeling studies suggest that adding smoking cessation interventions to lung cancer screening improves the cost-effectiveness of the latter by as much as 20 to 45 percent (Villanti et al., 2013). While not as cost-effective as smoking cessation alone, the cost-effectiveness of a combined screening and cessation program was superior to screening alone (McMahon et al., 2011). "Given the large number of estimated screening-eligible people who are current smokers, a small increase in cessation will have a very large public health benefit," Taylor stressed.

Many view lung cancer screening as another opportunity to counsel patients who smoke about smoking cessation and to offer them resources to aid their attempts to quit if they express an interest in them. "It can be a teachable moment," Hoffman said. He pointed out Park's study, which found those primary care providers who participated in the NLST and assisted and arranged follow-up for smoking cessation for screened patients were associated with higher quit rates among their patients (Park et al., 2015). "But most providers offer less intensive interventions, and that is not effective," he stressed. Even when smoking cessation and lung cancer screening are not synergistic, Lathan noted, "smoking cessation counseling is integral to the screening because as clinicians, we can use these teachable moments to talk to our patients and help them stop smoking. Tobacco cessation has to be an equal partner to screening and not an afterthought."

Ostroff added that the multiple potential encounters with clinicians during the screening process provide the opportunity to deliver tobacco cessation advice and treatment. But she agreed with Hoffman that undergoing screening alone is certainly not sufficient to create the kind of complex behavior change needed to stop using an addictive substance like tobacco.

Ostroff noted that the consensus among all guidelines is that lung cancer screening includes smoking cessation advice and treatment. She added that "although we know what works for tobacco cessation, we do not know what works best in the context of lung cancer screening." Studts pointed out that people eligible for lung cancer screening are an older population who have smoked for many years. "Sometimes there is pessimism about helping individuals who are long-term tobacco users to achieve cessation," he said. But he and Slatore pointed to several studies in the literature that support the efficacy of cessation interventions in this population (Chen and Wu, 2015; Isenberg et al., 2016; Zbikowski et al., 2012). However, Slatore noted that many of the long-time smokers who successfully quit underwent intense interventions and willingly chose to be in a study on smoking cessation, "which is not exactly reminiscent of what is going on in the real world." A study of Medicare beneficiaries that followed them serially found the quit rate among people who smoke declined by about one-third of one percentage point per year, so that a smaller proportion of the population are quitting every year, he added (Isenberg et al., 2016). "Lung cancer screening probably offers another opportunity to help us both find these patients and hopefully find ways to help them quit. We need to do more work to help active smokers in this age group," Slatore said.

Challenges in Implementation

Ostroff conducted a survey of site coordinators in lung cancer screening programs to identify the perceived challenges in delivering smoking cessation therapy. Most reported that patients were not motivated to quit and resisted cessation advice and therapy. Coordinators also reported not having enough trained staff and time to dedicate to these interventions, as well as a lack of confidence that they knew how to help patients quit smoking and the guidelines for doing so (Ostroff et al., 2015). Systems issues hampering delivery of smoking cessation therapy reported by the coordinators included a lack of on-site support for treating tobacco cessation or readily available resources or referrals for cessation, as well as a lack of tobacco treatment specialists, reimbursement, and limited contact with patients. "As a public health community, we can and should be able to provide training and technical assistance to address these barriers," Ostroff said.

Her study found that academically affiliated screening sites did not provide more extensive cessation counseling and treatment than community settings, nor was a larger site more likely to have more intensive cessation efforts. The only factor that was significantly linked to intense cessation treatment was making smoking cessation treatment an organizational priority.

Ostroff's study found that nearly all sites asked patients about their smoking habits and advised people who smoke to quit, but only about half of sites offered tobacco cessation counseling or self-help materials. Similarly, only about half referred people who smoke to a quit line or to on-site cessation services. Approximately one-third recommended cessation medicines. "We are really good at asking and advising about smoking practices because you cannot determine eligibility for the screening unless you are assessing tobacco use and thankfully there is a high degree of advice. But where things clearly become suboptimal in terms of quality of care is the degree of assistance given to patients to help them quit smoking," Ostroff said.

Offering smoking cessation services also decreased at repeat scans compared to what was offered at baseline. Tobacco dependence is a chronic relapsing condition that often requires multiple quit attempts, Ostroff noted. "So the fact that we are seeing marked decline in tobacco treatment with repeat scans is another red flag for work that needs to be done," she said. Smith added, "You have to be patient and offer the opportunity to quit in a relentless way." Park also stressed the importance of providing consistent smoking cessation messages, "because when providers are not consistent in delivering their messages and do not mention smoking cessation, patients often interpret it as not being important. So we should think about consistency across our messages to our patients."

Results of Cessation Efforts Linked to Screening Programs

Several workshop participants reported on the results of studies on smoking cessation programs linked to lung cancer screening programs, many of which seem to refute common beliefs and concerns about linking cessation to screening, including that informing people about their risk of developing lung cancer at the time of screening would foster efforts to quit smoking, that negative lung scans would reassure people who smoke and make them less inclined to quit, or that offering smoking cessation services along with screening would drive patients away from the screening. Instead, the studies found other psychological factors that should be considered when offering smoking cessation therapy.

Taylor reported on four randomized cessation intervention studies conducted within lung cancer screening programs that used in-person counseling on screening day, telephone counseling, a tailored Web-based intervention, or self-help Internet resources. Though all of these studies reported promising quit rates between 5 and 33 percent, none found significant differences among the groups that received the interventions and the groups that received no intervention, or more standard interventions, Taylor said (Clark et al., 2004; Ferketich et al., 2012; Marshall et al., 2016; van der Aalst et al., 2012).

Taylor also conducted a cessation intervention trial with current individuals scheduled to undergo lung screening who were randomized to receive a list of cessation resources (usual care), or six telephone counseling sessions with a trained telephone counselor, in addition to the cessation resource list. The telephone counseling sessions consisted of motivational interviewing for those not ready to quit, encouragement to consider using nicotine replacement therapy when appropriate, and encouragement to talk with their primary care clinician about medicines that can help them quit smoking. There was also discussion of their screening results and how quitting now would reduce the chance of having an abnormal result in the future, while refuting participants' misconceptions that a negative scan gave them a "clean bill of health" and minimized the need to quit.

This study found that after a 3-month follow-up period, 17 percent of those who received the telephone counseling had quit biochemically confirmed abstinence, compared to only 4 percent of those in the usual care arm. This preliminary evidence suggests telephone-based cessation intervention is feasible and efficacious in the lung cancer screening setting, Taylor said. "The best thing about this intervention is that it is scalable via existing quit lines, and potentially able to reach a large number of current smokers who are undergoing lung cancer screening," she stressed. But Taylor noted several limitations of the study, including its small size, short-term follow-up, and largely Caucasian population.

Kitts reported on a study at the Lahey Hospital Clinic that found that the smoking cessation rates of those who were screened for lung cancer were two to three times greater than that of the general population (Kitts et al., 2016). Studts commented that "even though we are not seeing dramatic intervention effects, these data are still consistently showing better than background spontaneous quit rates, so there is opportunity to leverage."

Risk Perception

A core concept of smoking cessation programs is the notion that educating patients who smoke about their risk of developing lung cancer will inspire them to quit smoking. Park conducted a study of patients undergoing lung cancer screening at eight NLST sites nationwide in which she surveyed people who smoke prior to their screening and 1 year later. She found that the screening experience did not appear to change participants' perceived risk of developing lung cancer or promote smoking cessation (Park et al., 2013). When she then interviewed a subgroup of 35 of these participants, she found that although they recognized lung cancer often was a death sentence and that smoking contributed to their risk of lung cancer, many downplayed that risk, citing other factors that influenced lung cancer risk or thought that the risk was exaggerated. Most did not report being worried about developing lung cancer. "The responses suggested that smokers avoid thinking or worrying about their risks," Park concluded, adding that they exhibited cognitive dissonance about their risk of lung cancer, or made other health behavior changes they thought might compensate for the effects of smoking on their risk of lung cancer. Although none of those interviewed had quit smoking, about half had reported they had cut back on smoking or made other health behavior changes, such as increasing their levels of exercise, that they thought would lower their risk of lung cancer. "They were making efforts at making a behavior change, but they were not successful because they did not have assistance," she said.

Park also reported on racial differences in risk perception. She said small studies have indicated that African Americans have a lower perceived risk of lung cancer. Other studies have found that African Americans have poorer cessation outcomes and are less likely to quit. Park conducted a study with participants from the NLST and found that although African Americans were more likely to make an attempt to quit smoking during the trial than Caucasians, they were less successful at smoking cessation. African Americans in the NLST were also significantly more likely to perceive their risk of developing lung cancer as lower than Caucasians (Kumar et al., 2016).

Impact of Screen Results on Willingness to Quit

Although lung cancer screening is seen as an opportunity to encourage smoking cessation in patients who smoke, some people at the workshop expressed concern that negative results from such screening might actually deter patients from quitting. As previously mentioned, data from the VA demonstration project found numerous misconceptions people have about lung cancer screening, with some patients thinking screening itself could protect them against lung cancer, or that they could be lucky smokers, meaning that despite smoking, they could be immune to lung cancers, as indicated by their negative scans, Hoffman said. Another study found some screened smokers reported being more relaxed and confident about their body after having a negative scan (Zeliadt et al., 2015). "There is some concern that the patient would see a negative scan as a license to smoke," Slatore noted. But he conducted a systematic review of patients in randomized clinical trials who underwent lung cancer screening and found that screening by itself does not affect smoking behavior, nor does it impact smoking cessation rates (Slatore et al., 2014). Park also reported on two studies which found that patients with repeated negative screening tests did not have a reduced likelihood of maintaining smoking abstinence or a higher likelihood of relapse after quitting smoking (Anderson et al., 2009; Clark et al., 2016).

Two screening trials have found that receiving a false-positive scan was linked to quitting smoking; the more suspicious the nodule detected was, the more likely people were to quit, Taylor reported (Tammemägi et al., 2014a; Taylor et al., 2007). Another study that followed screened patients for 4 to 14 years after trial enrollment found no relationship between screening results and quit rates (Barry et al., 2012). But Slatore noted that the population screened in all these trials is not representative of the general high-risk patients eligible for screening. He said that in interviews with patients who have incidentally detected (not detected through lung cancer screening) non-cancerous nodules in their lungs suggested that "real-world" patients are motivated to quit smoking, but more research among patients undergoing lung cancer screening is needed (Slatore et al., 2014).

The Importance of Empathy

Some experts expressed concern that aggressively pursuing cessation treatment during the lung screening process might drive away people who smoke. As Park said, "People are afraid that if they bring up smoking cessation, which is like the elephant in the room, that it would scare off patients." But she stressed that if counseling for smoking cessation is patient-centered and provides patients who smoke the opportunity to follow-up if they are interested in quitting, "we will not scare off anybody. And if we do not bring it up throughout the screening process, patients might hear that as permission to continue their behavior."

Taylor noted that in her study of a telephone counseling intervention for smoking cessation, which was provided after people participated in lung cancer screening, potential participants were explicitly told that they did not need to be ready to quit in order to participate. Many participants who had all six counseling sessions never set a quit date. "That was okay because we talked about how they may not be ready to quit, but what they were learning now may provide them with the skills and background they would need once they were ready to quit. That was really important to how we were able to accrue people, 50 percent of whom reported they were absolutely not ready to quit," she said.

To prevent disenfranchising participants by asking about their smoking, Studts suggested that clinicians counseling people who smoke be trained in how to do it in an empathetic way, such as motivational interviewing, and to avoid badgering or stigmatizing patients. "If we can help folks responsible for this to be trained at the highest level of evidence-based tobacco treatment, then we can get around that barrier and hopefully would be doing a much better job of integrating cessation treatment as a vital part of screening," he said.

Intensity of Smoking Cessation Programs and Quitting Success

Several presenters noted that the success of smoking cessation interventions embedded in lung cancer screening trials depends on how intensive they are. In one study, Slatore reported, some screened patients were given a brochure about smoking cessation, while others were offered a computerized questionnaire that gave advice about smoking cessation based on participants' answers to questions. Fewer than one-quarter of the patients given the questionnaire completed it, and there was no difference in the quit rate of the two groups, both of which involved relatively low-intensity interventions (van der Aalst et al., 2012). "Just offering smoking cessation information and expecting people to act on it is probably not likely to happen," Slatore stressed.

But another similar study of screened patients gave participants in one group prescriptions for smoking cessation medicine for 3 months and provided four telephone conversations with them that were at least 10 minutes long. Sixty-one percent of these patients completed the smoking cessation intervention. One year later, approximately 20 percent were still not smoking, a quit rate significantly higher than screened patients not given the intervention (Pozzi et al., 2015). "There is evidence emerging that high-intensity programs embedded within a lung cancer screening program may be the way to go," Slatore said. He noted other studies that have also found that the more intensive cessation programs are, the more likely they are to be successful. "It may not matter as much what the intervention was, but rather how intense it was," he noted (Fu et al., 2014; Parkes et al., 2008).

Park agreed and referred to the results of her study of NLST participants who received smoking cessation therapy from primary care providers. This study found that when clinicians merely used the traditional approach of asking, assessing, and advising patients who smoke about cessation, it did not affect their quit rates (Park et al., 2015). But when they assisted participants with their smoking cessation efforts and arranged for a follow-up visit to talk about them, these participants had greater quit rates (Park et al., 2015). "Having a conversation about smoking is not as effective as really intervening," she said. But she noted that participants who had lower educational attainment were less likely to quit smoking even after clinicians have provided assistance and arranged follow-up with a smoking cessation intervention.

Massetti asked how intense smoking cessation interventions need to be in order to be effective in people undergoing lung cancer screening. Ostroff responded, "We do not know yet how many components we need and how many sessions to optimize a quit rate, so I advocate for a scalable adaptive model of tobacco cessation treatment delivery that is based on a flexible notion of a clinical workflow that you can always add onto. We have to be realistic about the resources a screening site has and where different intensities of interventions can and should be offered. I am not sure these sites can really start with the Cadillac and be sustainable."

Taylor suggested that cessation therapy could be provided off site from where screening occurs. "We do not want to rely on screening sites that are already overworked and overburdened and trying to figure things out. Once lung cancer screening programs are more under way and able to take this on, then more of it could happen within the lung screening site," she said. Park agreed with both Taylor and Ostroff and added that the reality of providing optimal, intensive smoking cessation interventions may be altered by how much insurers reimburse for such interventions. "We do not have modes of paying for them right now," Park said. "We are funding them now with grants and philanthropy and I hope over time we are able to collect data showing efficacy, effectiveness, and cost-effectiveness of this work so that can change." But she added that with the advent of the ACA, tobacco cessation treatment is now reimbursable, and there are federal guidelines that define exactly what types of cessation treatments are covered. "These are woefully underutilized," she said. "There are unique opportunities now to put cessation treatment into place."

Studts pointed out that in the rural low-resource community where he works, funding is used to offer training for lung cancer screening program coordinators to increase the number of certified tobacco treatment specialists who are available on site. He noted that there are currently only four such certified individuals in the entire state of Kentucky. The screening program he is a part of currently has a low volume of people being screened, so it is not unreasonable to give the coordinator the added responsibility of providing tobacco cessation treatment, especially when there are no other available options to which patients can be referred. "When you are the only game in town, you have to do it as well as you can do it," he said.

Stoms responded by suggesting Studts and others in low-resource communities take advantage of tobacco cessation programs held by respiratory care departments or other departments in their same institutions offering the lung cancer screening. "Respiratory therapists are underutilized health care practitioners. They have a wealth of knowledge and are trained to do and speak about smoking cessation treatment. Most hospitals have at least one or two respiratory care practitioners on staff," she said. Stoms reported on a lung cancer screening program in Pennsylvania that was integrated into a preexisting smoking cessation program at a community hospital instead of the reverse. Patients served at this hospital have a lower socioeconomic status, she noted, and a greater proportion are African American. Participants in the smoking cessation program who qualify for lung cancer screening meet with a program facilitator who arranges for a shared decision-making visit with a radiologist at the hospital, who can refer them for the screening.

VALUE AND EFFICIENCY IN LUNG CANCER SCREENING

Another area of discussion was the value and cost of lung cancer screening. Roth described two types of economic evaluations for lung cancer screening: cost-effectiveness analysis and budget impact analysis. Cost-effectiveness analysis compares the relative values of different interventions in creating better health and/or longer life. Costs can be considered from the payer's perspective or from a societal perspective, if it captures all costs, he said. Effectiveness is usually calculated in quality-adjusted life years (QALYs), or the duration and quality of survival quantified in a single measurement. Cost divided by QALYs provides a cost-effectiveness value that can be compared to an alternate intervention's cost-effectiveness value (e.g., LDCT lung cancer screening versus no screening), in order to calculate an incremental cost-effectiveness ratio. Many stakeholders use approximately $100,000 as the incremental cost-effectiveness threshold, but Roth said that a range of $50,000 to $200,000 is often considered (Gold et al., 1996; Neumann et al., 2014).

Budget impact analysis does not place a value on an intervention, but rather evaluates its effect on a specific budget. It considers the expected changes in expenditures of a health care system after the adoption of new interventions. It compares two scenarios—one with the adoption of the new technology and another without it, analyzing the differences in terms of resource use and cost. The results are typically presented as total cost to the health care system or health plan. A budget impact analysis can also be calculated as the cost per member, per month by dividing the total cost by the number of planned members over the time of the analysis (Sullivan et al., 2014).

A cost-effectiveness analysis of lung cancer screening based on NLST results found it was $81,000 per QALY gained, which is considered to be a moderate value, Roth said. The cost was $52,000 for every life-year gained (Black et al., 2014). Importantly, Roth added that this analysis was based on the three annual rounds of screening that occurred during the NLST trial, and not on the potentially 25 years of annual screening that could occur for eligible patients.

However, Roth noted, the cost-effectiveness for lung cancer screening approached or exceeded $100,000 when

- Future health care costs beyond the scope of the trial duration were included;
- Costs for the screening examination, follow-up, or surgery were increased;
- Pessimistic expectations of survival with localized lung cancer were assumed; or
- Small reductions in quality of life related to positive screening results and a diagnosis of localized lung cancer were included.

Subgroup analyses also found that cost-effectiveness varied substantially according to gender, age, and smoking status (see Table 6). The screen-

TABLE 6 Incremental Costs According to Subgroups in Examining the Cost-Effectiveness of Screening with Low-Dose Computed Tomography in the National Lung Screening Trial

Characteristic	Number of Participants	Incremental Costs	Incremental QALYs	Cost per QALY
		U.S. $	QALY	U.S. $
Sex				
Male	31,446	1,683	0.0115	147,000
Female	21,856	1,557	0.0340	46,000
Age at entry				
55-59 years	22,773	1,541	0.0101	152,000
60-64 years	16,333	1,520	0.0320	48,000
65-69 years	9,504	1,900	0.0351	54,000
70-74 years	4,685	1,905	0.0163	117,000
Smoking status				
Former	27,643	1,661	0.0027	615,000
Current	25,659	1,601	0.0369	43,000
Risk of lung cancer				
First quintile	10,660	1,453	0.0086	169,000
Second quintile	10,661	1,454	0.0118	123,000
Third quintile	10,660	1,651	0.0061	269,000
Fourth quintile	10,661	1,672	0.0515	32,000
Fifth quintile	10,660	1,851	0.0354	52,000

NOTE: CT = computed tomography; QALYs = quality-adjusted life years in examining the cost-effectiveness of screening with low-dose CT in the NLST.

SOURCES: Roth presentation, June 21, 2016; From *The New England Journal of Medicine*, William C. Black, Ilana F. Gareen, Samir S. Soneji, et al, Cost-Effectiveness of CT Screening in the National Lung Screening Trial, 371, 1793-1802. Copyright © 2016 Massachusetts Medical Society. Reprinted with permission from Massachusetts Medical Society.

ing was more cost-effective for females than males, for younger people than older, and for current smokers as opposed to former smokers.

Roth also described a budget impact analysis of lung cancer screening for Medicare beneficiaries, which had a 5-year time horizon and assumed a gradual uptake of LDCT screening over that time period. Relying largely on NLST results, this analysis found that implementation of lung cancer screening would result in about a $6.8 billion increase in the Medicare budget over the 5 years of analysis, amounting to about $2.22 per enrollee, per month. The majority of the increase in expenditures is attributable to the screening cost itself, and not to the costs of diagnostic work-ups or cancer care (Roth et al., 2015), and is similar to mammography, Roth noted (Gross et al., 2013). "There is going to be increased expenditure . . . and Medicare needs to plan for that," Roth said. This projected increase is substantial, he stressed.

Roth noted that these analyses did not consider possible improvements of screening management protocols based on Lung-RADS, nor the potential impact of smoking cessation interventions. In addition, both analyses were based on outcomes at academic centers, so they may not translate to community practices. One study suggested that the false-positive rate seen in the NLST (26.6 percent) could have been reduced to 12.8 percent by following Lung-RADS criteria, Roth pointed out (Pinsky et al., 2015). Roth estimated that Lung-RADS criteria could potentially save Medicare $300 million over 3 years by reducing the number of false positives and subsequent diagnostic follow-up expenditures (Roth et al., 2016). "As new iterations of Lung-RADS and other protocols come out, we need to continue to look at these factors and figure out what the potential economic impacts are as well as the resource use implications," Roth said.

"If this plays out at a broader level, there could be other economic implications not in the direction we would hope," Roth said. For example, the degree of long-term adherence to lung cancer screening could also affect cost-effectiveness and budget analyses. Kim noted that a budget analysis for lung cancer screening in the VA found an initial round of screening could cost between $531 and $908 million. That is just for the first 11 months, she stressed, and with the analysis assuming all eligible participants could be screened at once, which is unlikely. "It is not a cheap endeavor by any means. It will cost hundreds of millions of dollars per year," Kim said.

Roth said that there are finite resources for health care so "even if we conduct a cost-effectiveness analysis and determine something to be high value, if we do not have the money to pay for it, we can still break our budget." Black raised the issue that without institutional support, shared decision making and lung cancer screening may not be self-sustaining in terms of revenue. Mazzone noted that lung cancer screening may increase revenue by bringing in more patients for other services beyond lung cancer screening, such as health consultations and the treatment of other cancers. More documentation and research are needed to assess the financial implications of lung cancer screening on institutions or practices, he added.

SUGGESTED AREAS OF RESEARCH

Several speakers highlighted areas of research that could improve lung cancer screening, such as examining how to best reach vulnerable populations who are likely to benefit from lung cancer screening, and the effectiveness of lung cancer screening in these individuals. Patricia Ganz, director of cancer prevention and control research at the University of California, Los Angeles Jonsson Comprehensive Cancer Center, suggested conducting more research that assesses what kinds of cognitive services and strategies can improve access and adherence to lung cancer screening. Mazzone agreed: "We need a better understanding of who makes choices and why, and how we can help them to make the choices that ultimately are best for them as individuals. I think we have an opportunity to study our groups who do not come to be screened and add to that literature," he said. Lathan stressed that data on Latinos at high-risk for lung cancer is especially lacking, including data that indicate where they were born, because "Latino" is a large and heterogeneous category. Smieliauskas added that he was only able to identify four in-depth and well-designed studies aimed at identifying lung cancer screening capacity needs of hard-to-reach populations. Smith noted, "No group is responsible for looking at the geography within a state and determining how we collectively are going to meet capacity needs." He added that if this was done routinely, it could help overcome health disparities in underserved areas. Smieliauskas said it would be useful to update his maps on capacity constraints on lung cancer screening, given the recent expansion of ACR-accredited lung cancer screening centers.

Aberle noted the challenges in enrolling minorities in clinical trials based on her experience with the NLST. Within the first 2 months of launching all its sites, about 25 percent of all enrollees at seven sites represented minorities. Although those sites maintained an enrollment of special populations above that of other sites, "we did not have in place the mechanisms to sustain this effort across to the end of accrual," Aberle said.

"We learned you have to start early if you want to enroll representative populations. Probably in order to be sustainable, those programs have to be embedded within the communities and have to take advantage of the physicians and the local medical centers where these individuals would be treated," she added.

Copeland pointed out that the Lung Cancer Alliance provides a structure for collaborative research in community settings. "We know there are a lot of evidence gaps and we are not going to get another NLST, but we have structures in place to figure out what is happening at the community level and how we can improve it for both patients and providers. There is a huge opportunity here we need to take advantage of," she said. Doria-Rose suggested studying how communication is occurring between patients and clinicians in lung cancer screening programs in order to minimize breakdowns in the process.

Roth suggested conducting economic evaluations of lung cancer screening using real-world data from community practices. New economic analyses are also needed when new protocols are implemented, such as Lung-RADS, he added. Roth said that there are methods in health economics that estimate the return on investment of future studies in order to prioritize the value of studies and allocate resources. This approach could be applied to lung cancer screening clinical trials. "It might show that a very costly trial could have an even bigger return," Roth said, adding "There are so many uncertainties about real-world community practice that there might be a number of relatively small and inexpensive observational studies that could be really high value. These types of analyses could be used to point out those key studies and move them forward."

Ostroff and other workshop participants suggested that there be more research on how to best integrate tobacco cessation programs into lung cancer screening programs. Studts pointed out that the NCI has initiated a new request for research proposals in smoking cessation and lung cancer screening in community practice. "We really need to assess best practices in this setting, in terms of cost per quit rate," Ostroff said. "What kind of implementation strategies are needed to both establish and maintain cessation treatment in real-world settings? All of us are coming from screening sites where we sort of know one way of doing things and we need to start thinking about the common principles of screening sites and use that knowledge to identify patient, provider, and system-level barriers and scalable smoking cessation interventions that can be used—if not one size fits all—one size fits most," she said.

WORKSHOP WRAP-UP

Massetti briefly summarized key discussions throughout the workshop. She noted that there was a lot of emphasis on the challenges of communicating the potential risks and benefits of lung cancer screening, to both patients and health care professionals. She added that the balance of those risks and benefits vary according to an individual's smoking history and other lung cancer risk factors, and those risks would be weighed differently by specific individuals. "Benefits and harms are not universal for all people, but vary according to cultural and individual factors and have to be embedded within an individual's understanding of what they find important in terms of benefits and their comfort with risks and harms," she said.

That is why shared decision making in the context of lung cancer screening is so crucial, Massetti stressed, and noted that "some of the country's greatest minds and experts in decision making are thinking about how to develop tools that can be disseminated and made available for patients. There are all kinds of challenges around implementing, reimbursing, and finding the time for shared decision making, but there is also a tremendous amount of opportunity because we are really trying our best to do it well and move beyond just checking the box [to document] that it happened." Shared decision making is reframing the goal for lung cancer screening, she added. "Instead of the ideal outcome being that everybody who is eligible is screened, we want the outcome to be having people be comfortable with the decisions they made, based on their values and their own levels of risk," she said.

A major challenge in lung cancer screening discussed at the workshop is consistently defining the eligible population, Massetti noted. She added that "we need to do a better job of measuring and tracking what happens when screening happens to people who are not within [the standard eligibility criteria]—what are the benefits and harms for people outside those boundaries?" Tied into determining eligibility for lung cancer screening is understanding the applicability of NLST results to the general population in the community, including underserved populations that were underrepresented in the trial but most at risk for developing lung cancer. Massetti noted that there was a lot of discussion about how to translate research into practice: "How can we use the NLST as a model, but yet also move beyond that and make the decisions that need to be made to implement lung cancer screening in other health care settings [that are] different from those that participated in the NLST study?"

Massetti reiterated that lung cancer screening is a process, not just a screening test, and quality has to be ensured for every step of that process, including eligibility determinations, shared decision making, image acquisition and interpretation, communication of results, and management of patients over time. "There are so many opportunities for things to go right or wrong throughout that spectrum," she stressed. Massetti concluded by noting that lung cancer screening is in its infancy. "As we are encountering implementation nationwide of lung cancer screening, we are in a different world compared to when mammography or colonoscopy became available. That is why it is important to continue to evolve the tools available to providers and their patients, as well as our evidence and decision making, and that we continue to iterate that process as well," she said.

REFERENCES

ACR (American College of Radiology). 2014. *Lung-RADS version 1.0 assessment categories.* http://www.acr.org/~/media/ACR/Documents/PDF/QualitySafety/Resources/LungRADS/AssessmentCategories.pdf (accessed August 29, 2016).

ACR. 2016a. *ACR BI-RADS Atlas.* http://www.acr.org/Quality-Safety/Resources/BIRADS (accessed September 30, 2016).

ACR. 2016b. Accredited facility search. http://www.acraccreditation.org/accredited-facility-search (accessed October 18, 2016).

ACS (American Cancer Society). 2016. *Cancer facts & figures 2016.* Atlanta, GA: American Cancer Society.

AHRQ (Agency for Healthcare Research and Quality). 2016. *Lung cancer screening tools.* https://www.effectivehealthcare.ahrq.gov/tools-and-resources/patient-decision-aids/lung-cancer-screening/decisionmaking-tool (accessed June 30, 2016).

Albain, K. S., J. M. Unger, J. J. Crowley, C. A. Coltman, and D. L. Hershman. 2009. Racial disparities in cancer survival among randomized clinical trials patients of the Southwest Oncology Group. *Journal of the National Cancer Institute* 101(14):984-992.

Albano, J. D., E. Ward, A. Jemal, R. Anderson, V. E. Cokkinides, T. Murray, J. Henley, J. Liff, and M. J. Thun. 2007. Cancer mortality in the United States by education level and race. *Journal of the National Cancer Institute* 99(18):1384-1394.

Anderson, C. M., R. Yip, C. I. Henschke, D. F. Yankelevitz, J. S. Ostroff, and D. M. Burns. 2009. Smoking cessation and relapse during a lung cancer screening program. *Cancer Epidemiology Biomarkers & Prevention* 18(12):3476-3483.

Bach, P. B., and M. K. Gould. 2012. When the average applies to no one: Personalized decision making about potential benefits of lung cancer screening. *Annals of Internal Medicine* 157(8):571-573.

Bach, P. B., L. D. Cramer, D. Schrag, R. J. Downey, S. E. Gelfand, and C. B. Begg. 2001. The influence of hospital volume on survival after resection for lung cancer. *New England Journal of Medicine* 345(3):181-188.

Bach, P. B., M. W. Kattan, M. D. Thornquist, M. G. Kris, R. C. Tate, M. J. Barnett, L. J. Hsieh, and C. B. Begg. 2003. Variations in lung cancer risk among smokers. *Journal of the National Cancer Institute* 95(6):470-478.

Barry, S. A., M. C. Tammemägi, S. Penek, E. C. Kassan, C. S. Dorfman, T. L. Riley, J. Commin, and K. L. Taylor. 2012. Predictors of adverse smoking outcomes in the Prostate, Lung, Colorectal and Ovarian Cancer Screening Trial. *Journal of the National Cancer Institute* 104(21):1647-1659.

Black, W. C., I. F. Gareen, S. S. Soneji, J. D. Sicks, E. B. Keeler, D. R. Aberle, A. Naeim, T. R. Church, G. A. Silvestri, J. Gorelick, and C. Gatsonis. 2014. Cost-effectiveness of CT screening in the National Lung Screening Trial. *New England Journal of Medicine* 371(19):1793-1802.

Borgmeyer, C. 2014. Evidence lacking to support or oppose low-dose CT screening for lung cancer, says AAFP. http://www.aafp.org/news/health-of-the-public/20140113aafplungcarec.html (accessed September 19, 2016).

Brenner, D. R., P. Boffetta, E. J. Duell, H. Bickeböller, A. Rosenberger, V. McCormack, J. E. Muscat, P. Yang, H.-E. Wichmann, I. Brueske-Hohlfeld, A. G. Schwartz, M. L. Cote, A. Tjønneland, S. Friis, L. Le Marchand, Z.-F. Zhang, H. Morgenstern, N. Szeszenia-Dabrowska, J. Lissowska, D. Zaridze, P. Rudnai, E. Fabianova, L. Foretova, V. Janout, V. Bencko, M. Schejbalova, P. Brennan, I. N. Mates, P. Lazarus, J. K. Field, O. Raji, J. R. McLaughlin, G. Liu, J. Wiencke, M. Neri, D. Ugolini, A. S. Andrew, Q. Lan, W. Hu, I. Orlow, B. J. Park, and R. J. Hung. 2012. Previous lung diseases and lung cancer risk: A pooled analysis from the International Lung Cancer Consortium. *American Journal of Epidemiology* 176(7):573-585.

Carter-Harris, L., D. P. Ceppa, N. Hanna, and S. M. Rawl. 2015. Lung cancer screening: What do long-term smokers know and believe? *Health Expectations.* doi: 10.1111/hex.12433.

Chen, D., and L.-T. Wu. 2015. Smoking cessation interventions for adults aged 50 or older: A systematic review and meta-analysis. *Drug and Alcohol Dependence* 154:14-24.

Clark, M. M., L. S. Cox, J. R. Jett, C. A. Patten, D. R. Schroeder, L. M. Nirelli, K. Vickers, R. D. Hurt, and S. J. Swensen. 2004. Effectiveness of smoking cessation self-help materials in a lung cancer screening population. *Lung Cancer* 44(1):13-21.

Clark, M. A., J. J. Gorelick, J. D. Sicks, E. R. Park, A. L. Graham, D. B. Abrams, and I. F. Gareen. 2016. The relations between false positive and negative screens and smoking cessation and relapse in the National Lung Screening Trial: Implications for public health. *Nicotine & Tobacco Research* 18(1):17-24.

CMS (Centers for Medicare & Medicaid Services). 2015. *Decision memo for screening for lung cancer with low dose computed tomography (LDCT) (cag-00439n).* https://www.cms.gov/medicare-coverage-database/details/nca-decision-memo.aspx?NCAId=274 (accessed June 30, 2016).

CMS. 2016. *Grandfathered health plan.* https://www.healthcare.gov/glossary/grandfathered-health-plan (accessed September 19, 2016).

Crawford, C. 2014. Medicare panel recommends against covering CT screening for lung cancer. *American Association of Family Physician News.* http://www.aafp.org/news/health-of-the-public/20140521medcacctrec.html (accessed September 20, 2016).

Earle, C. C., P. J. Neumann, R. D. Gelber, M. C. Weinstein, and J. C. Weeks. 2002. Impact of referral patterns on the use of chemotherapy for lung cancer. *Journal of Clinical Oncology* 20(7):1786-1792.

Echeverría, S. E., L. N. Borrell, D. Brown, and G. Rhoads. 2009. A local area analysis of racial, ethnic, and neighborhood disparities in breast cancer staging. *Cancer Epidemiology Biomarkers & Prevention* 18(11):3024-3029.

Edwards, F. H., I. Datta, J. D. Hunt, K. Stefan, C. G. Ball, E. Dixon, and S. C. Grondin. 2014. The impact of computed tomographic screening for lung cancer on the thoracic surgery workforce. *The Annals of Thoracic Surgery* 98(2):447-452.

Elwyn, G., A. O'Connor, D. Stacey, R. Volk, A. Edwards, A. Coulter, R. Thomson, A. Barratt, M. Barry, S. Bernstein, P. Butow, A. Clarke, V. Entwistle, D. Feldman-Stewart, M. Holmes-Rovner, H. Llewellyn-Thomas, N. Moumjid, A. Mulley, C. Ruland, K. Sepucha, A. Sykes, T. Whelan, and the International Patient Decision Aids Standards (IPDAS) Collaboration. 2006. Developing a quality criteria framework for patient decision aids: Online international Delphi consensus process. *British Medical Journal* 333(7565):417.

Elwyn, G., D. Frosch, A. E. Volandes, A. Edwards, and V. M. Montori. 2010. Investing in deliberation: A definition and classification of decision support interventions for people facing difficult health decisions. *Medical Decision Making* 30(6):701-711.

Ersek, J. L., J. M. Eberth, K. K. McDonnell, S. M. Strayer, E. Sercy, K. B. Cartmell, and D. B. Friedman. 2016. Knowledge of, attitudes toward, and use of low-dose computed tomography for lung cancer screening among family physicians. *Cancer* 122(15):2324-31.

Ferketich, A. K., G. A. Otterson, M. King, N. Hall, K. K. Browning, and M. E. Wewers. 2012. A pilot test of a combined tobacco dependence treatment and lung cancer screening program. *Lung Cancer* (Amsterdam, Netherlands) 76(2):211-215.

Fiscella, K., P. Winters, S. Farah, M. Sanders, and S. G. Mohile. 2015. Do lung cancer eligibility criteria align with risk among blacks and hispanics? *PLoS ONE* 10(11):e0143789.

Fu, S. S., M. van Ryn, S. E. Sherman, D. J. Burgess, S. Noorbaloochi, B. Clothier, B. C. Taylor, C. M. Schlede, R. S. Burke, and A. M. Joseph. 2014. Proactive tobacco treatment and population-level cessation: A pragmatic randomized clinical trial. *JAMA Internal Medicine* 174(5):671-677.

Gates, A., U. Ranji., and L. Snyder. 2014. Coverage of preventive services for adults in medicaid. The Kaiser Commision on Medicaid and the Uninsured. http://files.kff.org/attachment/coverage-of-preventive-services-for-adults-in-medicaid-issue-brief (accessed September 30, 2016).

Gierada, D. S., P. Pinsky, H. Nath, C. Chiles, F. Duan, and D. R. Aberle. 2014. Projected outcomes using different nodule sizes to define a positive CT lung cancer screening examination. *Journal of the National Cancer Institute* 106(11):dju284.

Gold, M. R., J. E. Siegel, L. B. Russell, and M. C. Weinstein. 1996. *Cost-effectiveness in health and medicine.* 1st ed. Cambridge, UK: Oxford University Press.

Gross, C. P., J. B. Long, J. S. Ross, M. M. Abu-Khalaf, R. Wang, B. K. Killelea, H. T. Gold, A. B. Chagpar, and X. Ma. 2013. The cost of breast cancer screening in the medicare population. *JAMA Internal Medicine* 173(3):220-226.

Grubbs, S. S., B. N. Polite, J. Carney, W. Bowser, J. Rogers, N. Katurakes, P. Hess, and E. D. Paskett. 2013. Eliminating racial disparities in colorectal cancer in the real world: It took a village. *Journal of Clinical Oncology* 31(16):1928-1930.

Healthwise. 2016. *Why shared decision making?* http://www.informedmedicaldecisions.org/shareddecisionmaking.aspx (accessed August 29, 2016).

Hoffman, R. M., A. L. Sussman, C. M. Getrich, R. L. Rhyne, R. E. Crowell, K. L. Taylor, E. J. Reifler, P. H. Wescott, A. M. Murrietta, A. I. Saeed, and S. I. Mishra. 2015. Attitudes and beliefs of primary care providers in New Mexico about lung cancer screening using low-dose computed tomography. *Preventing Chronic Disease* 12:150112.

Hoggart, C., P. Brennan, A. Tjonneland, U. Vogel, K. Overvad, J. N. Østergaard, R. Kaaks, F. Canzian, H. Boeing, A. Steffen, A. Trichopoulou, C. Bamia, D. Trichopoulos, M. Johansson, D. Palli, V. Krogh, R. Tumino, C. Sacerdote, S. Panico, H. Boshuizen, H. B. Bueno-de-Mesquita, P. H. M. Peeters, E. Lund, I. T. Gram, T. Braaten, L. Rodríguez, A. Agudo, E. Sánchez-Cantalejo, L. Arriola, M.-D. Chirlaque, A. Barricarte, T. Rasmuson, K.-T. Khaw, N. Wareham, N. E. Allen, E. Riboli, and P. Vineis. 2012. A risk model for lung cancer incidence. *Cancer Prevention Research* 5(6):834-846.

Humphrey, L. L., M. Deffebach, M. Pappas, C. Baumann, K. Artis, J. P. Mitchell, B. Zakher, R. Fu, and C. G. Slatore. 2013. Screening for lung cancer with low-dose computed tomography: A systematic review to update the U.S. Preventive Services Task Force recommendation. *Annals of Internal Medicine* 159(6):411-420.

Infante, M., S. Cavuto, F. R. Lutman, E. Passera, M. Chiarenza, G. Chiesa, G. Brambilla, E. Angeli, G. Aranzulla, A. Chiti, M. Scorsetti, P. Navarria, R. Cavina, M. Ciccarelli, M. Roncalli, A. Destro, E. Bottoni, E. Voulaz, V. Errico, G. Ferraroli, G. Finocchiaro, L. Toschi, A. Santoro, and M. Alloisio. 2015. Randomized study of lung cancer screening with spiral computed tomography. *American Journal of Respiratory and Critical Care Medicine* 191(10):1166-1175.

Iñiguez, C. E. B., K. W. Armstrong, Z. Cooper, J. S. Weissman, C. T. Ducko, J. O. Wee, M. P. Martinez, R. Bueno, M. T. Jaklitsch, and D. C. Wiener. 2016. Thirty-day mortality after lobectomy in elderly patients eligible for lung cancer screening, *The Annals of Thoracic Surgery* 101(2):541-546.

The International Early Lung Cancer Action Program Investigators. 2006. Survival of patients with stage I lung cancer detected on CT screening. *New England Journal of Medicine* 355(17):1763-1771.

Isenberg, J. Y., A. R. Quiñones, C. G. Slatore, W. C. Bryson, and S. M. Thielke. 2016. Trends in cigarette smoking and cessation among medicare managed care recipients, 2005-2012. *Addictive Behaviors* 58:155-160.

Kagawa-Singer, M., A. Valdez Dadia, M. C. Yu, and A. Surbone. 2010. Cancer, culture, and health disparities: Time to chart a new course? *CA: A Cancer Journal for Clinicians* 60(1):12-39.

Katki, H. A., S. A. Kovalchik, C. D. Berg, L. C. Cheung, and A. K. Chaturvedi. 2016. Development and validation of risk models to select ever-smokers for CT lung cancer screening. *JAMA* 315(21):2300-2311.

KFF (Kaiser Family Foundation). 2016. The coverage gap: Uninsured poor adults in states that do not expand Medicaid. http://kff.org/uninsured/issue-brief/the-coverage-gap-uninsured-poor-adults-in-states-that-do-not-expand-medicaid (accessed October 19, 2016).

Kitts, A. K. B., A. B. McKee, S. M. Regis, C. Wald, S. Flacke, and B. J. McKee. 2016. Smoking cessation results in a clinical lung cancer screening program. *Journal of Thoracic Disease* 8(Suppl 6):S481-S487.

Kovalchik, S. A., M. Tammemägi, C. D. Berg, N. E. Caporaso, T. L. Riley, M. Korch, G. A. Silvestri, A. K. Chaturvedi, and H. A. Katki. 2013. Targeting of low-dose CT screening according to the risk of lung-cancer death. *New England Journal of Medicine* 369(3):245-254.

Kumar, P., I. F. Gareen, C. Lathan, J. D. Sicks, G. K. Perez, K. A. Hyland, and E. R. Park. 2016. Racial differences in tobacco cessation and treatment usage after lung screening: An examination of the National Lung Screening Trial. *The Oncologist* 21(1):40-49.

Lathan, C. S., B. A. Neville, and C. C. Earle. 2006. The effect of race on invasive staging and surgery in non-small-cell lung cancer. *Journal of Clinical Oncology* 24(3):413-418.

Lathan, C. S., L. T. Waldman, E. Browning, J. Gagne, and K. Emmons. 2015. Perspectives of African Americans on lung cancer: A qualitative analysis. *The Oncologist* 20(4):393-399.

Lewis, J. A., W. J. Petty, J. A. Tooze, D. P. Miller, C. Chiles, A. A. Miller, C. Bellinger, and K. E. Weaver. 2015. Low-dose CT lung cancer screening practices and attitudes among primary care providers at an academic medical center. *Cancer Epidemiology Biomarkers & Prevention* 24(4):664-670.

Li, K., A. Hüsing, D. Sookthai, M. Bergmann, H. Boeing, N. Becker, and R. Kaaks. 2015. Selecting high-risk individuals for lung cancer screening: A prospective evaluation of existing risk models and eligibility criteria in the German EPIC cohort. *Cancer Prevention Research* 8(9):777-785.

Ma, J., E. M. Ward, R. Smith, and A. Jemal. 2013. Annual number of lung cancer deaths potentially avertable by screening in the United States. *Cancer* 119(7):1381-1385.

Marcus, P. M., E. J. Bergstralh, R. M. Fagerstrom, D. E. Williams, R. Fontana, W. F. Taylor, and P. C. Prorok. 2000. Lung cancer mortality in the Mayo lung project: Impact of extended follow-up. *Journal of the National Cancer Institute* 92(16):1308-1316.

Marshall, H. M., D. A. Courtney, L. H. Passmore, E. M. McCaul, I. A. Yang, R. V. Bowman, and K. M. Fong. 2016. Brief tailored smoking cessation counseling in a lung cancer screening population is feasible: A pilot randomized controlled trial. *Nicotine & Tobacco Research* 18(7):1665-1669.

Mazzone, P., C. A. Powell, D. Arenberg, P. Bach, F. Detterbeck, M. K. Gould, M. T. Jaklitsch, J. Jett, D. Naidich, A. Vachani, R. S. Wiener, and G. Silvestri. 2015. Components necessary for high-quality lung cancer screening: American College of Chest Physicians and American Thoracic Society policy statement. *Chest* 147(2):295-303.

McKee, B. J., J. A. Hashim, R. J. French, A. B. McKee, P. J. Hesketh, C. R. Lamb, C. Williamson, S. Flacke, and C. Wald. 2015. Experience with a CT screening program for individuals at high risk for developing lung cancer. *Journal of the American College of Radiology* 12(2):192-197.

McMahon, P. M., C. Y. Kong, C. Bouzan, M. C. Weinstein, L. E. Cipriano, A. C. Tramontano, B. E. Johnson, J. C. Weeks, and G. S. Gazelle. 2011. Cost-effectiveness of computed tomography screening for lung cancer in the United States. *Journal of Thoracic Oncology* 6(11):1841-1848.

McMahon, P. M., C. Y. Kong, B. E. Johnson, M. C. Weinstein, J. C. Weeks, A. C. Tramontano, L. E. Cipriano, C. Bouzan, and G. S. Gazelle. 2012. The MGH-HMS lung cancer policy model: Tobacco control versus screening. *Risk Analysis* 32:S117-S124.

The National Lung Screening Trial Research Team, D. R. Aberle, A. M. Adams, C. D. Berg, J. D. Clapp, K. L. Clingan, I. F. Gareen, D. A. Lynch, P. M. Marcus, and P. F. Pinsky. 2010. Baseline characteristics of participants in the randomized National Lung Screening Trial. *Journal of the National Cancer Institute* 102(23):1771-1779.

The National Lung Screening Trial Research Team, D. Aberle, A. Adams, C. Berg, W. Black, J. Clapp, R. Fagerstrom, I. Gareen, C. Gatsonis, P. Marcus, and J. Sicks. 2011. Reduced lung-cancer mortality with low-dose computed tomographic screening. *New England Journal of Medicine* 365(5):395-409.

NCQA (National Committee for Quality Assurance). 2016. *HEDIS & performance measurement*. http://www.ncqa.org/hedis-quality-measurement (accessed August 29, 2016).

NCI (National Cancer Institute). 2011. *Radon and Cancer*. https://www.cancer.gov/about-cancer/causes-prevention/risk/substances/radon/radon-fact-sheet (accessed September 30, 2016).

NCI. 2016a. *NCI dictionary of cancer terms*. https://www.cancer.gov/publications/dictionaries/cancer-terms (accessed September 19, 2016).

NCI. 2016b. *Patient and physician guide: National Lung Screening Trial*. https://www.cancer.gov/types/lung/research/NLSTstudyGuidePatientsPhysicians.pdf (accessed September 28, 2016).

NCI. 2016c. *SEER stat fact sheets: Lung and bronchus cancer*. http://seer.cancer.gov/statfacts/html/lungb.html (accessed June 30, 2016).

Nelson, H. D., K. Tyne, A. Naik, C. Bougatsos, B. K. Chan, and L. Humphrey. 2009. Screening for breast cancer: Systematic evidence review update for the U.S. Preventive Services Task Force. *Annals of Internal Medicine* 151(10):727-W242.

Neumann , P. J., J. T. Cohen, and M. C. Weinstein. 2014. Updating cost-effectiveness—The curious resilience of the $50,000-per-QALY threshold. *New England Journal of Medicine* 371(9):796-797.

NIH (National Institutes of Health). 2016. *Population-based Research Optimizing Screening through Personalized Regimens (PROSPR)*. http://healthcaredelivery.cancer.gov/prospr (accessed September 26, 2016).

Oken, M. M., W. G. Hocking, P. A. Kvale, G. L. Andriole, S. S. Buys, T. R. Church, E. D. Crawford, M. N. Fouad, C. Isaacs, D. J. Reding, J. L. Weissfeld, L. A. Yokochi, B. O'Brien, L. R. Ragard, J. M. Rathmell, T. L. Riley, P. Wright, N. Caparaso, P. Hu, G. Izmirlian, P. F. Pinsky, P. C. Prorok, B. S. Kramer, A. B. Miller, J. K. Gohagan, C. D. Berg, and Prostate, Lung, Colorectal, and Ovarian (PLCO) Project Team. 2011. Screening by chest radiograph and lung cancer mortality: The Prostate, Lung, Colorectal, and Ovarian (PLCO) randomized trial. *JAMA* 306(17):1865-1873.

Ong, M. B. H. 2014. Bach: LCA center certification untrustworthy; CISNET models don't match. *The Cancer Letter*. http://cancerletter.com/articles/20140509_5 (accessed September 20, 2016).

Ostroff, J. S., A. Copeland, S. P. Borderud, Y. Li, D. R. Shelley, and C. I. Henschke. 2015. Readiness of lung cancer screening sites to deliver smoking cessation treatment: Current practices, organizational priority, and perceived barriers. *Nicotine & Tobacco Research* 18(5):1067-1075.

Park, E. R., S. J. Japuntich, N. A. Rigotti, L. Traeger, Y. He, R. B. Wallace, J. L. Malin, J. P. Zallen, and N. L. Keating. 2012. A snapshot of smokers after lung and colorectal cancer diagnosis. *Cancer* 118(12):3153-3164.

Park, E. R., I. F. Gareen, A. Jain, J. S. Ostroff, F. Duan, J. D. Sicks, B. Rakowski, M. Diefenbach, and N. A. Rigotti. 2013. Examining whether lung screening changes risk perceptions: NLST participants at 1-year follow-up. *Cancer* 119(7):1306-1313.

Park, E. R., I. F. Gareen, S. Japuntich, I. Lennes, K. Hyland, S. DeMello, J. D. Sicks, and N. A. Rigotti. 2015. Primary care provider-delivered smoking cessation interventions and smoking cessation among participants in the National Lung Screening Trial. *JAMA Internal Medicine* 175(9):1509-1516.

Parkes, G., T. Greenhalgh, M. Griffin, and R. Dent. 2008. Effect on smoking quit rate of telling patients their lung age: The Step2quit randomised controlled trial. *British Medical Journal* 336(7644):598-600.

Pastorino, U., R. Boffi, A. Marchianò, S. Sestini, E. Munarini, G. Calareso, M. Boeri, G. Pelosi, G. Sozzi, M. Silva, N. Sverzellati, C. Galeone, C. La Vecchia, A. Ghirardi, and G. Corrao. 2016. Stopping smoking reduces mortality in low-dose computed tomography screening participants. *Journal of Thoracic Oncology* 11(5):693-699.

Patz, E. F., Jr., P. Pinsky, C. Gatsonis, J. D. Sicks, B. S. Kramer, M. C. Tammemägi, C. Chiles, W. C. Black, D. R. Aberle, and National Lung Screening Trial (NLST) Overdiagnosis Manuscript Writing Team 2014. Overdiagnosis in low-dose computed tomography screening for lung cancer. *JAMA Internal Medicine* 174(2):269-274.

Patz, E. F., Jr., E. Greco, C. Gatsonis, P. Pinsky, B. S. Kramer, and D. R. Aberle. 2016. Lung cancer incidence and mortality in National Lung Screening Trial participants who underwent low-dose CT prevalence screening: A retrospective cohort analysis of a randomised, multicentre, diagnostic screening trial. *The Lancet Oncology* 17(5):590-599.

Pennsylvania Department of Health. 2016. Lung Cancer Screening Toolkit. http://livehealthypa.com/health-team/professional-education/educational-toolkits/lung-cancer-screening-toolkit (accessed September 26, 2016).

Peto, J. 2012. That the effects of smoking should be measured in pack-years: Misconceptions 4. *British Journal of Cancer* 107(3):406-407.

Pinsky, P. F., and C. D. Berg. 2012. Applying the National Lung Screening Trial eligibility criteria to the U.S. population: What percent of the population and of incident lung cancers would be covered? *Journal of Medical Screening* 19(3):154-156.

Pinsky, P. F., D. S. Gierada, P. H. Nath, E. Kazerooni, and J. Amorosa. 2013. National Lung Screening Trial: Variability in nodule detection rates in chest CT studies. *Radiology* 268(3):865-873.

Pinsky, P. F., D. S. Gierada, W. Hocking, E. F. Patz, and B. S. Kramer. 2014. National lung screening trial findings by age: Medicare-eligible versus under-65 population. *Annals of Internal Medicine* 161(9):627-633.

Pinsky, P. F., D. S. Gierada, W. Black, R. Munden, H. Nath, D. Aberle, and E. Kazerooni. 2015. Performance of Lung-RADS in the National Lung Screening Trial: A retrospective assessment performance of Lung-RADS in the NLST. *Annals of Internal Medicine* 162(7):485-491.

Pozzi, P., E. Munarini, F. Bravi, M. Rossi, C. La Vecchia, R. Boffi, and U. Pastorino. 2015. A combined smoking cessation intervention within a lung cancer screening trial: A pilot observational study. *Tumori* 101(3):306-311.

Roth, J. A., S. D. Sullivan, B. H. L. Goulart, A. Ravelo, J. C. Sanderson, and S. D. Ramsey. 2015. Projected clinical, resource use, and fiscal impacts of implementing low-dose computed tomography lung cancer screening in medicare. *Journal of Oncology Practice* 11(4):267-272.

Roth, J. A., S. D. Sullivan, and B. H. L. Goulart. 2016. The potential clinical, resource use, and fiscal impacts of Lung-RADS to inform lung cancer screening in Medicare. *Value in Health* 19(3):A6.

Schoen, R. E., P. F. Pinsky, J. L. Weissfeld, L. A. Yokochi, T. Church, A. O. Laiyemo, R. Bresalier, G. L. Andriole, S. S. Buys, E. D. Crawford, M. N. Fouad, C. Isaacs, C. C. Johnson, D. J. Reding, B. O'Brien, D. M. Carrick, P. Wright, T. L. Riley, M. P. Purdue, G. Izmirlian, B. S. Kramer, A. B. Miller, J. K. Gohagan, P. C. Prorok, and C. D. Berg. 2012. Colorectal-cancer incidence and mortality with screening flexible sigmoidoscopy. *New England Journal of Medicine* 366(25):2345-2357.

Silvestri, G. A., J. Handy, D. Lackland, E. Corley, and C. E. Reed. 1998. Specialists achieve better outcomes than generalists for lung cancer surgery. *Chest* 114(3):675-680.

Sin, D. D., C. M. Tammemägi, S. Lam, M. J. Barnett, X. Duan, A. Tam, H. Auman, Z. Feng, G. E. Goodman, S. Hanash, and A. Taguchi. 2013. Pro-surfactant protein B as a biomarker for lung cancer prediction. *Journal of Clinical Oncology* 31(36):4536-4543.

Slatore, C. G., C.Baumann, M. Pappas, and L. L. Humphrey. 2014. Smoking behaviors among patients receiving computed tomography for lung cancer screening. Systematic review in support of the U.S. Preventive Services Task Force. *Annals of the American Thoracic Society* 11(4):619-627.

Smieliauskas, F., H. MacMahon, R. Salgia, and Y.-C. T. Shih. 2014. Geographic variation in radiologist capacity and widespread implementation of lung cancer CT screening. *Journal of Medical Screening* 21(4):207-215.

Stacey, D., F. Légaré, N. F. Col, C. L. Bennett, M. J. Barry, K. B. Eden, M. Holmes-Rovner, H. Llewellyn-Thomas, A. Lyddiatt, R. Thomson, L. Trevena, and J. H. C. Wu. 2014. Decision aids for people facing health treatment or screening decisions. *Cochrane Database of Systematic Reviews* (1):CD001431.

Studts, J. L., Byrne, M. M., and R. J. Thurer. 2012. A conjoint analysis of lung cancer screening decisions among individuals at-risk for lung cancer. Paper presented at the Conjoint Analysis in Health Care Conference. Orlando, Florida.

Sullivan, S. D., J. A. Mauskopf, F. Augustovski, J. Jaime Caro, K. M. Lee, M. Minchin, E. Orlewska, P. Penna, J.-M. Rodriguez Barrios, and W.-Y. Shau. 2014. Budget impact analysis—principles of good practice: Report of the ISPOR 2012 budget impact analysis good practice II task force. *Value in Health* 17(1):5-14.

Tammemägi, M. C., H. A. Katki, W. G. Hocking, T. R. Church, N. Caporaso, P. A. Kvale, A. K. Chaturvedi, G. A. Silvestri, T. L. Riley, J. Commins, and C. D. Berg. 2013. Selection criteria for lung-cancer screening. *New England Journal of Medicine* 368(8):728-736.

Tammemägi, M. C., C. D. Berg, T. L. Riley, C. R. Cunningham, and K. L. Taylor. 2014a. Impact of lung cancer screening results on smoking cessation. *Journal of the National Cancer Institute* 106(6):dju084.

Tammemägi, M. C., T. R. Church, W. G. Hocking, G. A. Silvestri, P. A. Kvale, T. L. Riley, J. Commins, and C. D. Berg. 2014b. Evaluation of the lung cancer risks at which to screen ever- and never-smokers: Screening rules applied to the PLCO and NLST cohorts. *PLoS Medicine* 11(12):e1001764.

Tanner, N. T., M. Gebregziabher, C. Hughes Halbert, E. Payne, L. E. Egede, and G. A. Silvestri. 2015. Racial differences in outcomes within the National Lung Screening Trial. Implications for widespread implementation. *American Journal of Respiratory and Critical Care Medicine* 192(2):200-208.

Taylor, K. L., L. S. Cox, N. Zincke, L. Mehta, C. McGuire, and E. Gelmann. 2007. Lung cancer screening as a teachable moment for smoking cessation. *Lung Cancer* 56(1):125-134.

Tramontano, A. C., D. F. Sheehan, P. M. McMahon, E. C. Dowling, T. R. Holford, K. Ryczak, S. M. Lesko, D. T. Levy, and C. Y. Kong. 2016. Evaluating the impacts of screening and smoking cessation programmes on lung cancer in a high-burden region of the USA: A simulation modelling study. *British Medical Journal Open* 6(2):e010227.

USPSTF (U.S. Preventive Services Task Force). 2013. Modeling report: Other supporting document for lung cancer: Screening. https://www.uspreventiveservicestaskforce.org/Page/Document/modeling-report/lung-cancer-screening (accessed September 28, 2016).

USPSTF. 2014. *Final recommendation statement: Lung cancer: Screening*. https://www.uspreventiveservicestaskforce.org/Page/Document/RecommendationStatementFinal/lung-cancer-screening (accessed September 19, 2016).

USPSTF. 2016a. *Evidence summary: Lung cancer: Screening*. https://www.uspreventiveservicestaskforce.org/Page/SupportingDoc/lung-cancer-screening/evidence-summary4#copyright-and-source-information (accessed September 19, 2016).

USPSTF. 2016b. Grade definitions. https://www.uspreventiveservicestaskforce.org/Page/Name/grade-definitions (accessed October 11, 2016).

van der Aalst, C. M., H. J. de Koning, K. A. M. van den Bergh, M. C. Willemsen, and R. J. van Klaveren. 2012. The effectiveness of a computer-tailored smoking cessation intervention for participants in lung cancer screening: A randomised controlled trial. *Lung Cancer* 76(2):204-210.

Villanti, A. C., Y. Jiang, D. B. Abrams, and B. S. Pyenson. 2013. A cost-utility analysis of lung cancer screening and the additional benefits of incorporating smoking cessation interventions. *PLoS ONE* 8(8):e71379.

Volk, R. J., and L. E. Foxhall. 2015. Readiness of primary care clinicians to implement lung cancer screening programs. *Preventive Medicine Reports* 2:717-719.

Volk, R. J., H. Llewellyn-Thomas, D., Stacey, and G. Elwyn. 2013. Ten years of the International Patient Decision Aid Standards Collaboration: Evolution of the core dimensions for assessing the quality of patient decision aids. *BMC Medical Informatics and Decision Making* 13(2):S1.

Walker, G. V., S. R. Grant, B. A. Guadagnolo, K. E. Hoffman, B. D. Smith, M. Koshy, P. K. Allen, and U. Mahmood. 2014. Disparities in stage at diagnosis, treatment, and survival in nonelderly adult patients with cancer according to insurance status. *Journal of Clinical Oncology* 32(28):3118-3125.

Welch, H. G., and W. C. Black. 2010. Overdiagnosis in cancer. *Journal of the National Cancer Institute* 102(9):605-613.

Wender, R., E. T. H. Fontham, E. Barrera, G. A. Colditz, T. R. Church, D. S. Ettinger, R. Etzioni, C. R. Flowers, G. S. Gazelle, D. K. Kelsey, S. J. LaMonte, J. S. Michaelson, K. C. Oeffinger, Y.-C. T. Shih, D. C. Sullivan, W. Travis, L. Walter, A. M. D. Wolf, O. W. Brawley, and R. A. Smith. 2013. American Cancer Society lung cancer screening guidelines. *CA: A Cancer Journal for Clinicians* 63(2):106-117.

Wiener, R. S., L. M. Schwartz, S. Woloshin, and H. G. Welch. 2011. Population-based risk for complications after transthoracic needle lung biopsy of a pulmonary nodule: An analysis of discharge records. *Annals of Internal Medicine* 155(3):137-144.

Wille, M. M., A. Dirksen, H. Ashraf, Z. Saghir, K. S. Bach, J. Brodersen, P. F. Clementsen, H. Hansen, K. R. Larsen, J. Mortensen, J. F. Rasmussen, N. Seersholm, B. G. Skov, L. H. Thomsen, P. Tonnesen, and J. H. Pedersen. 2016. Results of the randomized Danish Lung Cancer Screening Trial with focus on high-risk profiling. *American Journal of Respiratory and Critical Care Medicine* 193(5):542-551.

Williams, D. R., and S. A. Mohammed. 2009. Discrimination and racial disparities in health: Evidence and needed research. *Journal of Behavioral Medicine* 32(1):20.

Wilson, D. O., and J. Weissfeld. 2015. A simple model for predicting lung cancer occurrence in a lung cancer screening program: The Pittsburgh Predictor. *Lung Cancer* (Amsterdam, Netherlands) 89(1):31-37.

Wood, D. E., G. A. Eapen, D. S. Ettinger, L. Hou, D. Jackman, E. Kazerooni, D. Klippenstein, R. P. Lackner, L. Leard, A. N. C. Leung, P. P. Massion, B. F. Meyers, R. F. Munden, G. A. Otterson, K. Peairs, S. Pipavath, C. Pratt-Pozo, C. Reddy, M. E. Reid, A. J. Rotter, M. B. Schabath, L. V. Sequist, B. C. Tong, W. D. Travis, M. Unger, and S. C. Yang. 2012. Lung cancer screening. *Journal of the National Comprehensive Cancer Network* 10(2):240-265.

Yarnall, K. S. H., K. I. Pollak, T. Østbye, K. M. Krause, and J. L. Michener. 2003. Primary care: Is there enough time for prevention? *American Journal of Public Health* 93(4):635-641.

Yousaf-Kahn, U., N. Horeweg, C. van der Aalst, K. ten Haaf, M. Oudkerk, and H. de Koning. 2015. Baseline characteristics and mortality outcomes of control group participants and eligible non-responders in the NELSON lung cancer screening study. *Journal of Thoracic Oncology* 10(5):747-753.

Yousaf-Khan, U., C. van der Aalst, P. A. de Jong, M. Heuvelmans, E. Scholten, J.-W. Lammers, P. van Ooijen, K. Nackaerts, C. Weenink, H. Groen, R. Vliegenthart, K. ten Haaf, M. Oudkerk, and H. de Koning. 2016. Final screening round of the NELSON lung cancer screening trial: The effect of a 2.5-year screening interval. *Thorax* doi: 10.1136/thoraxjnl-2016-208655.

Zbikowski, S. M., B. Magnusson, J. R. Pockey, H. A. Tindle, and K. E. Weaver. 2012. A review of smoking cessation interventions for smokers aged 50 and older. *Maturitas* 71(2):131-141.

Zeliadt, S. B., J. L. Heffner, G. Sayre, D. E. Klein, C. Simons, J. Williams, L. F. Reinke, and D. H. Au. 2015. Attitudes and perceptions about smoking cessation in the context of lung cancer screening. *JAMA Internal Medicine* 175(9):1530-1537.

Appendix A

Statement of Task

An ad hoc committee will plan and host a 1.5-day public workshop to examine the current state of lung cancer screening, challenges to the clinical implementation of low-dose computed tomography screening for lung cancer, and potential policy actions to improve lung screening programs. The workshop will feature invited presentations and panel discussions on topics that may include

- Barriers to implementation of lung cancer screening and strategies to overcome these obstacles.
- Challenges and strategies for identifying populations eligible for and most likely to benefit from screening.
- Decision aids for health care providers and patients to support shared decision making regarding lung cancer screening, including considerations of the balance of benefits and harms of screening.
- Strategies to best provide smoking cessation support for current smokers in the context of lung cancer screening.
- Practical measures for state and national public health surveillance of lung cancer screening.
- Strategies to promote continuous quality improvement of screening programs and downstream care, including monitoring and reducing adverse outcomes or harms resulting from follow-up of false-positive screening results.

- The economics of lung cancer screening, including considerations of costs broadly defined, such as impact on quality of life and morbidity and mortality related to screening.
- Measurement of the impact of lung cancer screening (including morbidity and mortality) on those who are eligible based on the U.S. Preventive Services Task Force recommendation as well as those who are outside the recommended age and other criteria.

The committee will develop the agenda for the workshop sessions, select and invite speakers and discussants, and moderate the discussions. An individually authored workshop proceedings of the presentations and discussions at the workshop will be prepared by a designated rapporteur in accordance with institutional guidelines.

Appendix B

Workshop Agenda

June 20, 2016

7:30 am **Registration**

8:00 am **Welcome from the National Cancer Policy Forum**
Michael Caligiuri, The Ohio State University Comprehensive Cancer Center
National Cancer Policy Forum Chair

Overview of the Workshop
Greta Massetti, Centers for Disease Control and Prevention
Planning Committee Chair

8:15 am **Session 1: Overview of the Evidence, Policy, and Practice Issues in Lung Cancer Screening**
Moderator: Barnett Kramer, National Cancer Institute

Review of the Evidence for Benefits and Harms of CT Screening for Lung Cancer

- USPSTF Systematic Review
    - *Michael LeFevre, University of Missouri*

- ACS, ACCP, ASCO, NCCN Systematic Review
  - *Peter Bach, Memorial Sloan Kettering Cancer Center*

CMS Coverage of Lung Cancer Screening
- *Joseph Chin, Centers for Medicare & Medicaid Services*

Challenges of Implementation: The Primary Care Perspective
- *Richard Hoffman, University of Iowa*

Panel Discussion

10:15 am **Break**

10:30 am **Session 2: Considerations and Challenges in the Implementation of Lung Cancer Screening**
Moderator: Christopher Lathan, Dana-Farber Cancer Institute

Identifying High-Risk Populations for Screening: Risk Modeling—Current Ideas, New Developments, and Future Potentials
- *Martin Tammemägi, Brock University*

Guideline Development for Lung Cancer Screening
- *Douglas Wood, University of Washington*

Addressing Health Disparities in Lung Cancer Screening
- *Christopher Lathan, Harvard University*

Capacity Constraints and Geographic Variation in Access to Lung Cancer Screening
- *Fabrice Smieliauskas, University of Chicago*

Radiology Workload and Follow-Up Considerations
- *William Black, Dartmouth University*

Panel Discussion

12:45 pm **Lunch Break**

1:30 pm **Session 3: Essential Elements of Effective Lung Cancer Screening Programs**
Moderator: Robert Volk, MD Anderson Cancer Center

American College of Radiology Resources to Improve the Quality and Safety of Lung Cancer Screening
- *Ella Kazerooni, University of Michigan*

Veterans Health Administration Lung Cancer Screening Demonstration Project: Results and Lessons Learned
- *Jane Kim, VA National Center for Health Promotion and Disease Prevention*

Shared Decision Making for Lung Cancer Screening: Definitions, Models, and Strategies
- *Robert Volk, MD Anderson Cancer Center*

Supporting Informed Decision Making About Lung Cancer Screening
- *Jamie Studts, University of Kentucky College of Medicine*

Panel Discussion
- *Session speakers and Richard Hoffman, University of Iowa*

3:30 pm **Break**

3:45 pm **Session 4: Strategies for Incorporating Smoking Cessation in Screening Programs**
Moderator: Jamie Studts, University of Kentucky College of Medicine

Evidence for Smoking Behaviors and Cessation in Lung Cancer Screening
- *Chris Slatore, Oregon Health & Science University*

Screening and Resistance to Cessation Efforts
- *Elyse Park, Massachusetts General Hospital*

Assessment of a Telephone Counseling Smoking Cessation Intervention in the Lung Cancer Screening Setting: A Randomized Pilot Study

- *Kathryn Taylor, Georgetown University*

Readiness and Capacity of Screening Sites to Implement Smoking Cessation

- *Jamie Ostroff, Memorial Sloan Kettering Cancer Center*

Panel Discussion

5:40 pm **Wrap-Up Day 1**
Greta Massetti, Centers for Disease Control and Prevention

June 21, 2016

7:30 am **Registration**

8:00 am **Session 5: Health System Infrastructure Needs to Implement and Monitor Screening**
Moderator: Greta Massetti, Centers for Disease Control and Prevention

Patient Outcomes Related to Lung Cancer Screening

- *Denise Aberle, University of California, Los Angeles*
- *Peter Mazzone, Cleveland Clinic*

Cost-Effectiveness of Lung Cancer Screening

- *Joshua Roth, Fred Hutchinson Cancer Research Center*

Long-Term Follow-Up of Patients and Surveillance of Impact

- *V. Paul Doria-Rose, National Cancer Institute*

Panel Discussion

10:00 am **Break**

10:15 am **Session 6: Stakeholder Reactions and Perspectives**
Moderator: Dan Sullivan, Duke University School of Medicine

- *Ide Mills, Patient Advocate*
- *Amy Copeland, Lung Cancer Alliance*
- *Kelly Latimer, Naval Hospital Pensacola*
- *Joanna Stoms, Pennsylvania Department of Health*
- *Robert Smith, American Cancer Society*
- *Steven Blumenfrucht, Aetna*
- *Peter Mazzone, Cleveland Clinic*

Panel Discussion

11:30 am **Workshop Wrap-Up**
Greta Massetti, Centers for Disease Control and Prevention

11:45 am **Adjourn**

Appendix C

Glossary

Coinsurance–the percentage of costs of a covered health care service that a patient is responsible for once the deductible has been paid (HealthCare.gov, 2016).

Decision aids–tools used to facilitate a shared decision-making conversation between a patient and clinician. These tools can help patients understand the clinical evidence and help them identify their preferences. Decision aids do not advise people to choose one option over another; instead, they help prepare patients to make informed decisions aligned with their values and preferences (Healthwise, 2016).

False negative–a person who has a disease but receives a negative test result.

False positive–a person who does not have a disease but receives a positive test result.

Incidental findings–clinical findings that are identified during diagnostic testing but are not related to the diagnostic test result (for lung cancer screening, this could include cardiac abnormalities, chronic obstructive pulmonary disease, aneurysms, or masses in other tissues).

Lead-time bias–an overestimation of a patient's survival benefit among individuals without symptoms who are screened for cancer, compared to individuals with cancer that are detected by signs and symptoms when survival is measured from the time of diagnosis (American College of Physicians, 1999).

Length-time bias–an overestimation of a patient's survival duration among individuals without symptoms who are screened for cancer due to the disproportionate number of slowly progressing cancers that will be detected (American College of Physicians, 1999).

Number needed to screen–the number of people who need to be screened to prevent one bad outcome.

Overdiagnosis–when a condition is diagnosed that would otherwise not go on to cause symptoms or death (Welch and Black, 2010, p. 605).

Pack-year–a way to measure the amount a person has smoked over a long period of time. It is calculated by multiplying the number of packs of cigarettes smoked per day by the number of years the person has smoked. For example, 1 pack-year is equal to smoking 1 pack per day for 1 year, or 2 packs per day for half a year, and so on (NCI, 2016).

Positive predictive value–the probability that individuals with a positive test result actually have the disease. True Positives/(True Positives + False Positives)

Screening–checking for disease when there are no symptoms. Because screening may find diseases at an early stage, there may be a better chance of curing the disease (NCI, 2016).

Sensitivity–the proportion of people with a disease who are correctly identified from all positive test results for the disease. True Positives/(True Positives + False Negatives)

Shared decision making–is a collaborative process that allows patients and their providers to make health care decisions together. It takes into account the best clinical evidence available, as well as the patient's values and preferences. Shared decision making is not a goal. The goal is better health decisions to achieve outcomes that matter most to the patient. And shared decision making is a way to reach that goal. A proven process to incorporate the patient's voice in health care decisions, shared decision making is the pinnacle of patient-centered care (Healthwise, 2016).

Specificity–the proportion of people who are correctly identified as not having a disease from all negative test results for the disease. True Negatives/ (True Negatives + False Positives)

REFERENCES

American College of Physicians. 1999. *Finding and redefining disease.* http://ecp.acponline.org/marapr99/primer.htm (accessed September 30, 2016).

HealthCare.gov. 2016. *Coinsurance.* https://www.healthcare.gov/glossary/co-insurance (accessed September 30, 2016).

Healthwise. 2016. *Why shared decision making?* http://www.informedmedicaldecisions.org/shareddecisionmaking.aspx (accessed August 29, 2016).

IOM and NRC (Institute of Medicine and National Research Council). 2001. *Mammography and beyond: Developing technologies for the early detection of breast cancer.* Washington, DC: National Academy Press.

NCI (National Cancer Institute). 2016. *NCI dictionary of cancer terms*. https://www.cancer.gov/publications/dictionaries/cancer-terms (accessed September 19, 2016).

Welch, H. G., and W. C. Black. 2010. Overdiagnosis in cancer. *Journal of the National Cancer Institute* 102(9):605-613.